C000225883

Master your Mind
Befriend your Body

First published 2014 by Hummingbird Effect
an imprint of Upfront Publishing of Peterborough, England.

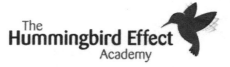

www.fast-print.net/store.php

MASTER YOUR MIND
BEFRIEND YOUR BODY
Copyright © Denise Collins 2014

ISBN: 978-178456-113-0

All rights reserved

No part of this book may be reproduced in any form by photocopying
or any electronic or mechanical means, including information storage
or retrieval systems, without permission in writing from both the
copyright owner and the publisher of the book.

The right of Denise Collins to be identified as the author of this work has
been asserted by him in accordance with the Copyright, Designs and
Patents Act 1988 and any subsequent amendments thereto.

A catalogue record for this book is available from the British Library

An environmentally friendly book printed and bound in England by
www.printondemand-worldwide.com

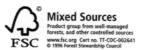

Mixed Sources
Product group from well-managed
forests, and other controlled sources
www.fsc.org Cert no. TT-COC-002641
© 1996 Forest Stewardship Council

PEFC Certified
This product is
from sustainably
managed forests
and controlled
sources
www.pefc.org

This book is made entirely of chain-of-custody materials

– MASTER YOUR MIND –
– BEFRIEND YOUR BODY –

– DENISE COLLINS –

Introduction

Mastering your mind is crucial to maximising your potential in terms of success, happiness and fulfilment in any and all areas of your life. Your mind is both your most valuable ally and potentially your most dangerous opponent. The truth is that these days many people spend more time learning to understand the applications of their smartphone than they do the capabilities of their own mind. Mastering your mind is the art of realising that the circumstances of your outer world are, at least in part, the creation of your inner world. This realisation can be remarkably empowering for some people and more than a little scary for others.

Befriending your body is a way of connecting with your physical self that will free you from the insidious influence of the multi-billion dollar industries which are built on the need for you to be unhappy with who you are. In place of self-loathing because you are too fat, or too thin, or too old or (..... fill in the appropriate blanks) instead you can begin to create true individual body esteem. The harsh reality is that for the vast majority of people the ideal image of what your physical appearance should be is always going to be unattainable. Therefore to pursue it is to be doomed to failure and misery. This is exactly what these industries rely upon to make profit. What if, instead of hating and punishing yourself for not being able to fit the ideal, you learn to genuinely appreciate, work with and improve the real body that you actually have?

Mind Body And…?

Although spirit or soul is not specifically mentioned in the title of this book, the thinking behind *Master Your Mind Befriend Your Body* is holistic in the sincerest sense. People have minds and think but we are more than just our thoughts. We have physical bodies, but that is not all that we are. We are at our very core, soul or spirit or personality or essence, however you choose to describe that part which is neither mind nor body yet flows though all of it.

Please let me briefly explain what *Master Your Mind Befriend Your Body* is all about and how it will benefit you. In the 21st century we have become overwhelmed with choice and variety to the extent that sometimes it seems impossible to choose for fear of making the wrong choice. We are totally overloaded with information and the rate and pace of technological change has created an almost alien environment where we have seemingly endless opportunities available to us, yet most people are less fulfilled than ever. We have lost touch with the importance of basic concepts such as cause and effect, and the reality that our actions have consequences. We have been brainwashed into having expectations of quick fixes, rewards without the necessity to strive and success without skill. There is an epidemic of wasted minds that are out of control, dangerously unruly and in need of mastery to be used optimally. There is widespread dissatisfaction among all age groups and both sexes with our physical bodies. Even if our bodies are healthy and in perfect working order it is common to think of them as somehow not good enough, ugly or loathsome. Many people neglect or actually damage their physical bodies either consciously or through ignorance. Each and every one of us is a unique individual. That is a biological fact of our DNA. It is now thought by scientists that even in identical twins, which have the same DNA, that they have it in very slightly different configurations. You are a totally unique individual simply because no one else has lived your life.

No one else has experienced all of everything you have experienced and all the resulting thoughts and feelings and decisions that came about because of those experiences. Each of us follows a unique path. You are not here by accident. There is a purpose to your life, even if you are not yet fully aware of it. Therefore I am interested not only in accompanying you on your path to personal (and/or professional) development, so that you can enrich various areas of your life such as wealth and work, love and relationships, health and wellbeing. I am also keen to help you go beyond this into an exploration of the transpersonal. In very basic terms the various disciplines of psychology developed along the lines of Psychoanalytical, the idea that we are products of our past. Behavioural, that outward behaviour can be modified by conditioning and thereby the experience of the person changes as a result. Humanistic with a focus on understanding human existence in terms of areas such as the self, health, hope, love, creativity, being, becoming individuality, meaning and self actualisation. To Transpersonal, which seeks to integrate the individual personal, spiritual and transcendent. I hope that you will find discovering *Master Your Mind Befriend Your Body* or MMBB for short, a fulfilling and exciting journey that can bring true authentic alignment and a focus on qualities such as responsibility, cooperation, love, meaning and purpose. A journey that can truly allow you access to inner guidance and wisdom in order to transform your inner world and your outer reality.

Master Your Mind

Denise Collins

One
Is there nothing really new?

I f you think that the idea that your thoughts create your reality all started with Bärbel Mohr and *The Cosmic Ordering Service* in 1995 or Rhonda Byrne and *The Secret* in 2006, think again. The idea that the way we think can help us manifest health, wealth and happiness goes back a bit further than that. In the first century Greek Stoic philosopher Epictetus said, "Men are disturbed not by things, but by the view they take of them." In 1841, Ralph Waldo Emerson, American essayist, lecturer, poet and leader of the Transcendentalist movement of the mid-19th century wrote, "every man in his lifetime needs to thank his faults" and "acquire habits of self-help" as "our strength grows out of our weakness". In 1859, Samuel Smiles, author and government reformer, published *Self-Help*. The opening sentence is: "Heaven helps those who help themselves". In 1902, James Allen, philosophical writer, published *As a Man Thinketh*, "a man is literally what he thinks, his character being the complete sum of all his thoughts." In the early 19th century in the USA the New Thought Movement developed. The idea of new thought, or higher thought as it is sometimes known, promotes the idea that infinite intelligence or God is supreme, universal, everlasting, everywhere in all real things and people. The New Thought Movement says that divinity dwells within each of us as spiritual beings and thought can be used as a force for good. It proposed that our mental states are carried forward into manifestation and become our experience in daily living. Sound familiar? In 1906, William Walker Atkinson who was an attorney, merchant, publisher, occultist and an American pioneer of the New Thought Movement, wrote and published *Thought Vibration or the Law of Attraction in the Thought World*. In 1907, Elizabeth Towne, writer and editor, published Bruce MacLelland's book *Prosperity Through Thought Force*, in which he summarised the "Law of Attraction" as a New Thought principle, stating, "You are what you think, not what you think you are." In 1910 Wallace Delois Wattles, an American author, wrote *The Science of Getting Rich*. In 1936 Dale Breckenridge Carnegie produced *How to Win Friends and Influence People*. In 1937 Napoleon Hill, New Thought author wrote *Think and Grow Rich* describing the use of repeated positive thoughts to attract happiness and wealth by tapping into an "infinite Intelligence". I hope that this brief glance in the direction of history shows that the idea of mastery of the mind creating results in the real world is not some new-age, pixie dust nonsense.

Positive thinking for pessimists. In the 21ˢᵗ century some psychological, self-help approaches almost browbeat us into believing that we should think only positive happy thoughts. Indeed, we may be made to feel like failures or frauds if we cannot achieve a perpetually positive state of mind. Ready for a somewhat revolutionary idea? Good, here goes then. Negative thinking is not bad. It is natural. The ability to think the worst is arguably, in fact, essential for the very survival of the human race. I believe that the notion of totally positive thinking is quite frankly stupid. Just as totally negative thinking is stupid. Nothing is ever all totally good or all totally bad. To live life is to experience ups and downs. To deny this and attempt to reframe or put some positive spin on every experience is not only inauthentic but also reduces the richness of real life to a mere parody of itself.

Thoughts are powerful. Perhaps beyond measure. Yet just because you think something, does not make it so. Negative thoughts are not the problem. It is the act of totally believing your negative thoughts that can be problematic. A significant aspect of mastering your mind is the realisation that you are not your thoughts and that your thoughts are not even necessarily accurate. So a good starting point to mastering your mind is to dispense with the notion that what you are thinking is good or bad, true or false, positive or negative and instead to decide how useful a particular thinking style is. Developing the ability to think in new ways even in old situations is powerfully liberating. Training yourself to expand your awareness and broaden your focus of attention to begin to notice more of what there is to notice will develop your ability to master your mind.

Mindfulness has become somewhat of a buzz term in the fields of psychology and personal development. Mindfulness awareness originates from Buddhist meditation. But as far back as 1979 Jon Kabat Zinn was developing mindfulness as a secular practice with his "mindfulness based stress reduction" programme at the University of Massachusetts medical centre. MBSR was a fusion of mindfulness meditation and cognitive behavioural therapies (CBT). Some regard mindfulness as a set of skills that can be learned, some as more of a mental state, some see it as a training of awareness. Whatever you choose to call this, a focus on present moment awareness of thoughts, feelings, bodily sensations and the immediate environment rather than ruminating about the past or imagining the future, of acceptance of thoughts rather than judgment of them, is an effective pathway to mastering your mind.

Full Mind For many of us, for much of the time our minds are full. Right now the rapid rate and pace of progress and change we are expected to keep up with is simply unprecedented in human history. Many people experience mental overwhelm as a result of overload from technological and entertainment devices designed to make life easier and keep us amused. With the advent of mass instant communication and the internet, it has become increasingly challenging to differentiate between information and opinion. Being on 24/7 input means we have no opportunity to "fire gaze" as our ancestors would have done. And little time to just be with our thoughts, without external stimuli, in order to have the time to process events in the way that even our parents' generation had.

How does your garden grow?

Any process of development could be likened to gardening. Creating a lovely garden takes more than throwing a handful of seeds on the ground and hoping for the best. The first stage is to assess the ground, the area in its current state, as it is. Being realistic, not seeing it as better than it is nor worse than it is, but as it is. Then comes the job of clearing the ground of debris and weeds. This requires action not just thinking about what needs to be done. What are you holding on to? What is holding you back?

Once the ground is clear it is time to plan, to envision the garden of your dreams. After the planning comes the planting of what you want to grow. Remembering that we often overestimate what can be done in the short term but underestimate how much we can do in the long term. Once we have planted, we need to nurture and nourish. Our efforts combined with a little help from Mother Nature allow the garden to grow.

Time then, to enjoy it, while keeping in mind that gardens, like life, are all about seasons and cycles. Nothing lasts for ever and the weeds will once again take over if not kept in check. Life is about ups and downs. If nothing lasts, then there is no need to dwell on the bad because that won't last. And you must remember to enjoy the good because it too won't last.

Master your mind and Befriend your body and you can literally transform your life. This can be the making of you. Improve your inner world and you will improve the results you get in the outer world.

So, would you like a really simple formula for getting whatever you want in life?

You would? Ready? Here goes.

Really simple formula for getting whatever you want in life:

Decide what you want and then do whatever needs to be done in order to achieve it.

Okay, it isn't profound, but you have to admit it is simple.

So what's preventing you?

At this point you may well be asking something along the lines of, "well if it is really that simple, what gets in the way?"

Well the **first** issue is that while this formula may be simple, (aka uncomplicated), simple is not the same as easy (aka requiring no effort).

The **second** is that while we often know what we don't like, or don't want, we can still be unclear about exactly what it is we do want. Sometimes what we want is not simply the opposite of what we don't want. So maybe you have never given enough energy to actually defining what you want in achievable terms. The focus has been in the wrong place preventing you from seeing what may be obvious.

Then there is the little matter of how **complex** we human beings are. The truth is that we usually want lots of different things, all at the same time. And often these various desires are in conflict with each other. So it can feel as if the path towards our goals is a case of: one step forward two steps back.

Another issue is that what we think we want is sometimes really more about what we think getting something will actually mean to us if we get it! So it isn't really what we want at all, but rather a means that we hope will get us what we actually want. For example, someone might say that what they want is to lose weight. But underlying this is the belief, hope or assumption that being a certain waist measurement, BMI or physical weight will automatically result in something else, e.g. feelings of happiness or confidence, a better relationship or love life. So in this example, in fact the real goal or desired outcome is happiness, confidence, a better relationship or love life, rather than actual weight loss. The weight loss is merely a perceived means to an end. While improving your relationship to your body is essential for true total wellbeing, you don't have to be Britain's next Top Model, or Arnold Schwarzenegger to achieve healthy balance.

Fears and Wants

Our innate primitive need for survival has us constantly, unknowingly reacting to these two basic fears:

1. Fear of rejection. At some level we all have a need to be accepted as a "part of the tribe". This is innate and necessary for our very survival. Some people talk of a self-limiting "fear of success" but in truth this is really just a fear of being judged by others and ultimately rejected.
2. Fear of failure. Humans need to have an innate aversion to risk, again in order to survive. The safest option is to repeat the known, to do the same things in the same way. Trying something new which may potentially lead to making a mistake could be fatal.

Our innate primitive need for survival is reflected in the two basic wants that drive much of our lives:

1. The desire for acceptance and love. We are not solitary creatures therefore we crave social acceptance and have a deep need to give and receive affection.

2. The desire for success. Human beings are programmed to progress. We have a desire to move in the direction of improvement. From the basics like our environment and material possessions to self-actualisation and self-individuation. Throughout psychological schools of thought and philosophy the move towards the transpersonal is evident. We all at some level strive to give our existence purpose and meaning.

What does this all mean? Human beings are meaning makers and problem solvers. To put it simply, we cannot not think. It is important to identify what things mean to you, because meaning has an impact even if you are not consciously aware of it. Once you have made conscious that which was previously unconscious you have choice and therefore more power.

For what purpose do I want X? Purpose is important in order to distinguish between end goals and means goals. For example, I may say that what I want is money. But if I assess for what purpose I want it, what having money will actually give to me, get for me or do for me, I will uncover the real deeper desire. This may be to feel secure or achieve freedom. The end goal is therefore actually security or freedom. Money is only one way that I have identified to perhaps achieve this. Money therefore is not the end goal. It is a means to a desired end. Unless I address this, it is possible that I might acquire money but still feel insecure or trapped. After all, how much is enough? And what happens if I lose it or someone takes it? Understanding the underlying purpose of a desire empowers you to find additional ways to achieve your end goals. In the above example, it doesn't mean that I have to abandon my goal of making money it just means I understand more deeply why it is of importance to me.

In what ways is this important? What makes this important to me?

Importance is connected to our sets of beliefs and values. Beliefs and values are what motivate us. They are also how we evaluate our actions. Unless the importance of a goal is understood it is unlikely to happen. There is always some ambivalence to any change. Unless the importance is clearly established, then taking the required action will be much more difficult. In order to gain something it may mean that you have to give something up.

What kind of person do you want to be? What kind of person do you have to be to achieve this? Does the outcome or goal fit with your identity? During *Master Your Mind Befriend Your*

Body we will look at issues of identity and explore the idea that we are all made up of competing sub-personalities or differing aspects to what constitutes who we are.

21st century challenges

The time we live in is what it is; both wonderful and terrible. Progress brings with it new problems and challenges for human beings who have not evolved that much in thousands of years. 21st century living is in many ways detrimental to human beings. Why? Because human beings still have fairly basic primitive physical bodies and minds, but we are attempting to operate in an almost alien environment which has progressed and changed much more rapidly than most people have. MMBB will explore the idea that much of the progress of the 21st century actually represents an environment that is detrimental to our psychological, physical and emotional health and wellbeing. More and more people are increasingly living unconsciously, inhabiting lives that they are part of yet disconnected from.

Physical and mental wellbeing. In the "developed" world, obesity is regarded as a disability that requires sympathy and treatment; depression and stress are seen as simply inevitable aspects of modern day life to be managed with solutions created, at a cost, by pharmaceutical companies. Although most people would now acknowledge as common sense the fact that our minds and bodies are inextricably linked, many of us still behave as if they are not. There may be a tendency to focus on developing one while ignoring the other. There seems to be an ever-increasing epidemic of people who not only do not take care of their bodies, but who actually hate and despise them. Imbalances in either mind or body can be reflected in the other. You are your body, but it is not you. You are your mind but that isn't all that you are. Many people seem to have lost touch with basic concepts like life cycles and cause and effect. Instead, engaging in the quest for perfection, immortality and everlasting youth through fads or short cut measures.

Looking in the wrong place. Many people spend a lot of time and energy seeking external solutions to what are essentially internal problems. The assumption is that being, doing or having more / better / bigger of the latest version of something will make a difference to how we feel psychologically on the inside. We have lost the ability to use our innate intuition and tune into our own internal resources and abilities. Instead seeking external answers to internal challenges.

Information overload. Unprecedented access to information on a 24/7 basis is now taken for granted. In an environment of advanced social media and open access internet, it is becoming increasingly challenging to distinguish between what is true fact and what is merely conjecture or opinion. Essentially, between what is information and what is misinformation.

Want or need? The absurdity is that the richer the developed world becomes, the less satisfied, the less content, the less happy many people are. It is as if the more we have, the more we think we need, or at least the more we want. It can be easy to persuade ourselves that our wants are actually needs. Because we are constantly shown images of other people who have more, no matter how much we attain there is always more to want.

Boredom. The paradox is that too much freedom can result in boredom, because when you are free to decide exactly whatever you want to do then everything can become unappealing. If you get your life to the point where it is totally secure, certain and there are no risks involved in anything, then this too can result in boredom. And boredom in the 21st century can be very dangerous as there is a plethora of unhealthy ways to entertain ourselves.

Not good enough. It is not unusual for even highly "successful" people to experience a sense of somehow not being quite good enough. Or feeling like a fraud, who will someday be found out. If we feel that we are not good enough, we are likely to project an image of what we believe is good enough, rather than being who we truly are.

Two
What do you really want?

In an age that has spawned many personal and professional development systems, we are encouraged to set goals and go for what we want. However, for many people the core problem goes something like: "How can I begin to decide what I want, when I don't even know who I am?"

Who are you?

Until the little matter of identity is sorted out, goals are difficult to establish let alone pursue. We have unprecedented ways to constantly compare ourselves, our lives, our achievements, with others. And often the feeling is that somehow we don't measure up. Sometimes it seems that we have been hijacked by an ever-increasing obsession with short-term pleasure in place of longer term satisfaction. Quick fixes in place of genuine solutions and hedonistic instant gratification rather than true happiness.

What is the main reason for doing anything or everything?

What is the most significant desire most people have at their very core, which drives everything else? What is it that if we perceive it to be missing nothing can fill the void?

Happiness. Not the short-term distractions it can be tempting to settle for, but deep inner happiness. The state may be known by many labels: peace, wellbeing, satisfaction, fulfilment. Whatever you choose to call it, we each know it when we experience it. It is possible that at the core, any goal or ambition can be reduced to the simple desire to be happy. Think of the old trio of health, wealth and happiness. If you had to make a choice, which do you consider is most important to you? How important is even health if you are unhappy? How many perfectly fit and healthy people commit suicide or sabotage their lives because they are unhappy? How many people who have money, who could even be considered wealthy, are still unhappy and no amount of material fortune can shift that? These things are, of course, important. And often it is not until we lose them that we realise just how significant they are. But consider for a moment, would you rather be happy even if you don't have wealth? Would you rather be healthy but not be happy? For those who have found it is possible to achieve the elusive state of real happiness, they are able to deal with everything else. Anyway, the gist of the idea is that if you want something in your life to change, you have to be prepared to actually do something different. As the now familiar saying goes, if you always do what you have always done, you will continue to get what you have always got.

You are here

At some time or another, perhaps if you have been lost or trying to find your way in an unfamiliar place, you must have come across one of those maps with a big arrow accompanied by the words "you are here". This is a nice metaphor because in order to improve anything you need to assess the current situation. Awareness and acceptance of what is, is a necessary starting point for any change. Taking some time to pause, to reflect, to not just listen but to hear, to not merely look but to see in order to notice and understand where you are now can be very useful. For some people even the thought of contemplating their life without the interruption of external distractions can be frightening. But it is the only way to reconnect to your own self. To connect to real sources of your own inner personal power, wisdom and strength.

To begin to plan how to direct your attention and actions toward what is important, to what really matters, what does the present moment mean to you? What does it require, need or demand? And how does this align with your longer term goals, plans and desired outcomes? Of course, the future is not certain and some might say that the very act of looking towards the future can change it. However, you need to have identified a desired destination when setting out on a journey. Unless, that is, you are happy to go round in circles or eventually end up somewhere you don't want to be.

Attend to the basics first.

You need a strong foundation or else everything that is built on it will wobble. This is true of personal development also. The basics need to be in place. If you are hungry and don't know where your next meal is coming from you are unlikely to be very engaged with ideas of personal growth. Until the basics for survival are in place there is unlikely to be energy for much else. If your life is falling apart it may not be the best time to embark on a journey of self-improvement. You need to learn how to swim before deciding to do it alone across the Channel. If you are currently going through some tough stuff and have picked up this book searching for some support, help or inspiration on how to make your life better, then I sincerely commend you for wanting to take control and help yourself. Already, just by doing this, you have set yourself apart and you have demonstrated that you are not a victim. Even if life has been or is harsh at present you are not a victim. No matter how tough things are in this moment you are ahead of the game. However, if stuff is happening for you currently there is a slightly different set of strategies that I would like to offer you that might be more time-relevant to you right now before you push yourself too hard too fast and try to move through all the ideas and actions in the rest of this book. You will still benefit from reading the book but I would strongly recommend that you consider the ideas and suggestions offered here in this section before expecting too much of yourself at this particular time in your life.

For a long time psychology focused on pathology, on what is wrong with people and why. In more recent times attention has turned towards the study of resilience. This is described in many different ways. One of the best definitions in my opinion is that resilience is a deep sense of knowing that, whatever is happening, you can get through the current conditions of your life and therefore you can see beyond this moment. This means that no matter how hard things are you do not have to be totally overwhelmed by the present moment and whatever is happening right now.

In any endeavour you require strength to achieve progress. You cannot train physically at your best if you are injured or lacking in energy because you are not eating the right food. And you cannot expect yourself to develop emotionally or psychologically if you have an emotional injury that needs time and the appropriate attention to heal properly. I am all for encouraging you to push yourself beyond what you perhaps believe you can do. But all in good time. Maybe at the moment your focus needs to be on getting back in good shape. Whatever is happening, however bad things are, you can still be grateful in the moment for what there is in your life you are appreciative of and thankful to have. It does not mean that you have to be happy / positive or that you can't or should not be sad about the stuff that isn't the way you want it. You see, it is all about balance. Now I know that might not sound that sexy or radically exciting, however, I really think that balance is very underrated when it comes to the human experience. Fulfilment often is the result of a good job done well rather than the manic highs and lows of super achievers. It might sound a bit odd but times of stress, unhappiness or trauma can be the best times to really examine your default patterns of thinking, feeling and behaving. Any personal limitations you have made part of your identity can become very apparent. After all, it is supremely easy to think about personal development when life is jogging along and we are not really personally challenged. I once heard Tony Robbins say that we should, "Define the game in win-able ways". I think this is very pertinent in terms of facing challenges in life. Basically, make sure you are not setting yourself up for failure by focusing on the stuff that you cannot alter or influence. If times are tough for you for whatever reason at the moment, give yourself credit and the time and space to heal.

Really, in truth, I suppose this section is applicable to everyone and anyone who is reading this book because even if it does not apply to you right now, the fact is that the conditions of our life can change dramatically in less than a heartbeat. We can be going along on our merry way thinking everything is fine and dandy with the world and BAM! something happens. So even if this section is not at present relevant to you it could be good to be aware of it as a resource that is available should you need it in the future. We sometimes make things more complicated than they need to be. It is a simple fact that if you are in pain you need to identify the real source and work out what it means to you. And then set about focusing on healing it.

Success often originates from the ability to have and exercise good judgement so that we make good decisions. And the ability to do this often actually comes from learning gained via experience. Which isn't always good or positive. Sometimes the very best learnings eventually come about as a result of the worst experiences. The only way we can actually learn how to be resilient is to go through hard times. You can't come up with an answer to a question you have not yet been asked. None of us can truly know how we will react in a given situation until we are actually there.

If you are going through pain in your life at the moment of whatever type, I truly, sincerely do feel for you and it is my fervent hope that I can help you in some way. We all go through painful experiences and it is my belief that if we go through pain and do not learn anything from it, even if the learning is that we can survive and that we are resilient even if we don't recognise it at the time, then that is tragic because it is likely that we may be doomed to be hurt by the same thing in the same way again. Learning to manage your state or developing an optimistic or positive attitude does not make you immune from ever experiencing pain or feeling down, sad, hurt or unhappy. It just means that you know that it won't last for ever and be all pervasive in every part of your life. It does not have to define your identity or the entire story of your life.

Some personal development approaches appear to offer techniques that can change emotional states instantly, no matter what is going on in your life. These approaches can lead to people feeling guilty or as if they have failed if they cannot do this. In reality, a positive attitude or mindset is far more powerful and useful than positive thinking. To be able to learn from life events and truly believe that it's not what happens to you, it is what you think about what happens to you that is significant, maybe true, however, all things have an appropriate timescale.

If you are having financial problems there is no use sticking your head in the sand like the proverbial ostrich and thinking positive thoughts while you use a credit card to buy a place on a personal development course. You need to assess the situation and take whatever sensible action is necessary. If you are in poor health. deciding that all you need to do is think happy thoughts could potentially prove fatal if it is all you do. If you are emotionally hurting you may need time to heal. So if stuff is going on for you at the moment the priority must be to ensure your security and safety.

I worked with a client, Sheila, who came for coaching because her 20-year marriage had ended suddenly. Sheila was devastated as she had always considered her husband her best friend. They also ran a business together. The end of the relationship meant she lost everything. Her well-meaning friends encouraged her to start dating. Not surprisingly, given her vulnerable state, she fell into a relationship with a totally unsuitable person. This new man chipped away at her already low confidence. Sheila had always believed in personal development and started berating herself for not being able to focus on the positives and get on with making a new start. If someone is drowning they need to be thrown a life ring. It is not the right time to start training for a cross-Channel swim. Sheila was in a bad way because the pain was all still current. Sheila had been trying to force her recovery but at best she temporarily put a *Band-Aid* over a severed artery.

In this scenario, first she needed to stop and take stock. This would provide her with the opportunity to accept the elements of the situation she had no control over and to identify what she did have control over. Rather than rushing to find some way to avoid the pain, she needed to decide what she actually wanted, giving herself the opportunity to experience the full range of her emotions; from sadness to anger. The end of any relationship is like bereavement and requires an appropriate time period to grieve. If her husband had died her friends would probably have accepted her need to grieve and would not have encouraged her to get "back out on the dating scene" to find an immediate replacement. A new relationship at that point with everything else going on would at best be a temporary distraction. However, her desperation to not face the pain of the break-up made her a target that attracted an unhealthy relationship with the wrong type of person.

Stress overloads the brain with powerful hormones that are intended only for short-term emergency situations. Prolonged periods of stress can increase the levels of cortisol in the bloodstream and create many negative effects such as impaired cognitive performance. So stress literally makes us stupid. We are not able to make good decisions when stressed. Other effects include: suppressed thyroid function; blood sugar imbalances such as hyperglycaemia; decreased bone density; decrease in muscle tissue; higher blood pressure; lowered immunity and inflammatory responses in the body; slowed wound healing, and other health consequences. Stress has even been linked to increased abdominal fat, which is associated with a greater amount of health problems than fat deposited in other areas of the body.

So it is wise to think safety and security first. Only when you are well emotionally, physically and mentally can you really make the most of any personal development work. The idea that it is somehow possible (or even desirable) to be perfectly happy all of the time and live lives totally devoid of any kind of discomfort or pain without anything ever going wrong is crazy. To be human is to feel as well as to think. The aim of a good life is not to NOT feel. It is to be able to deal with our human emotions. You are less likely to appreciate the sun in a climate where it never rains. You don't experience happiness or contentment if you are never unhappy because it would be just a flat-line life. A grey zone of okay-ness.

Three
Who are you? = the past.

I n order to choose your goals, ambitions and desired outcomes, you may first have to discover a little more about who you actually are and what is of real importance to you. When you discover who you are, you can decide who you actually want to be. A good way to begin this process of self-exploration is to take a look back at where you came from in order to examine your personal past. I am not proposing that any of us are a total product of our history. I do not believe that we enter the world as completely blank sheets shaped totally by our experiences. However, the past, chapter one of your life, is important. It is where you gained those first experiences that shaped how you initially learned to view yourself, the world and other people. Exploring your past is not an exercise in looking for a scapegoat or excuses. It is useful only if it leads to greater awareness and understanding which can empower you to be, to do and to have what you want in the present and the future. The truth is that whether your past was good, bad or indifferent, it is over. If you had a great past, you are blessed. If you had a past filled with trauma and unhappiness then what is of real importance is what you do with that fact.

As a child you were dependent upon your caregivers and accepted their view of the world as all that existed. Although to some extent we all carry this early view with us, as you grow, mature and make your own way in the world as an independent adult you get to choose your opinions and beliefs. Our early background, our family history and childhood experiences create a foundation for the adults we become. It does not determine completely who we are destined to be but it is useful to consider these early influences.

Put aside some time to consider your past. Perhaps gather some old photographs of you as a child and important people, creatures or places that had some significance or impact on you growing up. Arrange to talk to an older family member or a parent to ask about what life was like for them when you were a child. Consider your early influences then take some time to write or record what you learned to expect from:

- the world,
- other people,
- yourself?

When you have finished, without blame or criticism, consider if these ideas are still useful or helpful to you now in terms of creating the life you want?

Make two lists, one for any positive messages (e.g. "anything is possible") and one for any that may hold you back or hinder your progress in the present, (for instance, "you could do better").

Use Your Past Usefully

Find ways to remind yourself of everything that was positive and create ways to build on your strong foundation. Create ways to finish any "unfinished business" that may be a hangover from your past which is preventing you from fully experiencing the present and creating your desired future. You do not have to minimise or deny anything that happened in your past but now is the time to move on from it. It happened. Learn from it or be victim of it. You have a choice to be empowered or defeated.

Four
Who are you? = the present.

Who are you and who do you want or aspire to be?

Recently I was running a training course during which we looked at the importance of identifying our values. It was so interesting to realise that even though values have such a fundamental impact, not only on who we are, but also on whether we are happy and fulfilled, or frustrated and miserable, yet they can seem really difficult to define and elusive.

One participant actually asked, 'If my values are so important, why do I find it so hard to know what they are? Shouldn't I be able to just naturally reel them off?'

Another participant asked how our values differed from our opinions?

Another wondered what the difference is between beliefs and values?

And everyone wanted a method for beginning to identify, explore and then implement their values more, so they could live a more authentic, congruent life.

Our values are the ideas that we believe to be important. They act as a guide to the choices we make and determine our priorities. They influence the plans that we make and how we like to spend time. They provide us with a way to evaluate if our decisions and actions are in accordance with what we consider important. If this is the case we are likely to feel satisfied, content and happy. If not, the opposite may be true and we may feel frustrated, discontented and unhappy.

Our opinions and beliefs are both based upon and reveal our values. For example, if you express an opinion like, "I think it is really important to be upfront with people", this probably reveals that honesty is one of your values. If someone tramples on your values, it hurts. This is because they are important and implicit, therefore there is an inherent assumption that if something is important to us, it should be held in the same high regard by everyone else.

It may not feel like an easy task but it is well worth taking the necessary time to identify your personal values. Because whether or not you consciously recognise them they still have an influence in your life.

Here Is A Relatively Simple Exercise To Help You Identify Your Values.

1. List the various areas of your life. What actually constitutes your life?
   For example, Finance, Career, Relationships, Love, Health, Wellbeing, Purpose & meaning beyond the personal. Of course, you may identify additional areas or feel that some of the above do not apply to your life.
2. Select an area that is very important (if possible the MOST important to you).
3. What are your values in this area?
   List your top 10
   For example, honesty, hard work, loyalty, doing your best, being successful, caring for others. These are merely examples. Decide what is of importance to you in this area.
4. Reduce this list by half.
5. How do you actually "do" or live these values? Think of some specific examples of how you live according to, say, honesty.
6. Look again at these values and decide if they also apply to any of the other areas of your life? For

example, if you have chosen family, do the same values also apply to work?

7. If you were to attempt to live even more closely according to your values is there anything you would need to stop doing, start doing, do more of or do less of?

8. What would be the opposite of 7.?

9. Which is closer to your current reality, 7 or 8?

10. How could what you have noticed during this exercise assist you with being more "you" and living a life that is closely aligned to what is important to you?

Our values could be considered to be a bit like a guiding compass because we use them consciously and unconsciously to direct us towards what is of importance to us. And also to retrospectively evaluate our actions. If we are behaving in alignment with our values we experience peace and contentment. If, for whatever reason, our actions are in conflict with our values, we will feel inauthentic and ill at ease. Values can be thought of as "important concepts" e.g. honesty, loyalty, freedom. Some values will be present across all contexts and could be described as core values. Others will be more secondary and may come to the fore in various situations.

Beliefs are essentially opinions or assumptions. A feeling that something is so, even if the feeling is irrational and there is no actual proof. We often act as if our beliefs are irrefutable facts. Beliefs can be divided into two basic types: those that limit us and those that empower us. So perhaps rather than struggling to establish whether a belief is true or false, right or wrong, it may be better to ask how useful is this belief in this given situation? Our personality, what constitutes our very identity, could be regarded as how we express and apply our values and beliefs.

Until You Truly Value Yourself No One Else Can.

This sounds like such a stock phrase which is seen on posters and quoted so frequently. But think about it for a moment. So many people do not even begin to recognise, let alone fulfil their true potential simply because they undervalue themselves.

If you do not value yourself, anyone else who tries to will be proved to be a bad decision maker. This is basically because if you do not value yourself you can't value anyone else who tries to value you. Why would you?

Until you value yourself you may neglect and abuse your body and let others do the same. Why would you not?

Internal External Referencing

If you undervalue yourself you will not rate your own opinions. So you will look outside of yourself for guidance and validation. If you do not value yourself, you will see no value in what you think, so you will always regard your thoughts and ideas as less important than those expressed by others. This is potentially very dangerous because it leaves you open to manipulation and abuse. Especially as the way that some people attempt to hide their own insecurities and feelings of inadequacy is by belittling or looking down on others. I like the quote that says: "the only time you should ever look down on anyone is when you are offering them a hand up…".

What Is The Source Of The Pain You Are Trying Not To Feel?

Undervaluing yourself is destructive. Some people turn their feelings of inadequacy outwards and try to control or destroy others. And some people turn this inwards and self-destruct by various means. They may disregard their own safety and welfare by indulging in reckless activities. They may attempt to self-medicate with drugs, alcohol or even food. This can provide a short-term quick fix. However, bigger and more frequent doses are required. Some people then see this symptom of self-medication as the actual problem. So they give themselves a hard time about their addictions or lack of willpower. They may attempt to refrain, but without addressing the underlying cause this is unlikely to be sustainable long term. Think about it, in successful rehab programmes participants are not merely told to "stop" the behaviour. It is not as simple as just stop doing that. The hole in the soul that the person is attempting to fill needs to be identified and healed.

In the 21st century it is as if we consider that the only thing worthy of value is perfection. However, I am human and humans are rarely perfect. My life is real and real life is rarely perfect. Anyway, I think that perfect is overrated because where is there to go if you are there already?

Denise Collins 2014

A True Story

If each and every being on this planet is unique, an individual, quite literally one of a kind (which is not the same thing as being perfect) in what ways do we learn to undervalue ourselves?

I would like to share what I believe to be an exquisite real life example of how it is possible that the process of learning to undervalue ourselves does not have to be the result of abuse or neglect in childhood. Even in the most loving, indulgent, permissive families the message that somehow you are not as important as someone or something else can be implicit.

In full blown, very animated, loud, three-year-old style my granddaughter was explaining to me the intricacies of the game she was playing, while at the same time I was attempting to have a "grown-up" conversation with my son, her father.

'Wait a minute,' I said to her, 'I am just talking to daddy.'

In less than a heartbeat she replied, 'Yes I know, and I am talking to you.'

I think this is a lovely example of how often we inadvertently give the message that other people or things or activities are more valuable or somehow more important. Think about it, "I am just conversing with someone else rather than you....; I am just watching the TV...; I am just doing the ironing....; I am just...... just......"

The Answer?

Sorry, but there really is no one easy quick fix solution that will work for every person. However, it is useful to remember that if you do undervalue yourself you have probably been doing this for a long time. And when we do anything for a long time we tend to get good at it. So rather than seeking a magic wand solution, recognise that you have probably developed your ability to undervalue yourself over a long period and using a drip-drip effect, while consciously or unconsciously seeking evidence to confirm your beliefs about how you are not good enough or not as good as…

This awareness is essential because, quite simply, until we are aware of something we are not in a position to change it. Engaging with and perhaps even sharing some of the ideas and exercises in this book is a great start. Developing the ability to value yourself is a journey and every step is important. Here are 6 suggestions:

- Stop comparing yourself. It is pointless because it is highly likely that there will always be someone "better".
- Embrace the fact that you are you and no one else. You are the only example of you, so logically this makes you the perfect example of you. Perfect in all your imperfections as a human being. As Oscar Wilde said, 'Be yourself everyone else is already taken.'
- Get over yourself! Or rather step outside of yourself and do a realistic evaluation. Take some time to identify your strengths and play to them. We are too often encouraged to ignore our talents and focus energy instead on improving what we are not very good at. When you were a child this was useful to ensure that you at least had an opportunity to make improvements. But as an adult it is just a plain waste of time which is likely

to achieve little except to reinforce the tendency to undervalue yourself.

- Recognise your achievements. Even if you feel like these are not that great (e.g. "If I could achieve that, it can't be that difficult"..... Groucho Marx, "I don't want to belong to any club that will accept people like me as a member"). Some people who undervalue themselves actually have a fear of being considered arrogant if they acknowledge their talents. However, there is a significant difference between arrogance and confidence. Confidence about competence can never be arrogance.

- Valuing yourself is not about being better than. If you value yourself you will find it easier to value others. This creates equality, a win-win rather than one-upmanship.

- Develop the ability to be self-aware and to reflect on how you can improve. But do not engage in self-criticism. Accept personal responsibility for and understanding of the effect of others on you and the effect you have upon others.

I can be strong because I recognise my weakness

I understand joy because I know despair

I acknowledge that I am good enough because I realise I have flaws

I possess wisdom because I learn from experience

I will never be perfect because I am a human being

Denise Collins 2014

Five
Who could, might, can, will you be in the future?

D *iscover who you are then decide who you want to be in order to create the life you desire.*

So you have looked at the past and the present and now it is time to begin to plan the future. The future is a wonderful place which is full of opportunities and experiences that you can't even begin to imagine yet because they haven't happened. The future is open and fresh and new and untouched.

Just as when you are preparing for a journey, a trip or a holiday you do not pack everything you own. You decide what to take with you and what to leave behind. So too this is the case with preparing for your journey into the future. You don't have to take your entire past and present with you. You can decide to take into your future only what is useful, helpful and beneficial. Everything else you can simply decide to leave behind.

Each Of All Of Everyone Of Me.....

In psychology there are various ideas about the concept of competing sub-personalities. Not split personalities of "The Three Faces of Eve" archaic idea of schizophrenic multiple personalities battling for supremacy. But rather a more rational, normal concept that postulates that what constitutes our identity is a complex thing. Can anyone of us really truly state that they have one single unchanging "I" who they are in every situation, with every person, all of the time? Or are we made up of a collection of different parts? Perhaps you refer to these as different sides or aspects of yourself. These various characters may come to the fore and be either helpful or unhelpful in different situations. Understanding and engaging with this idea may make achieving goals easier. For example the sub-personality that really wants to get healthier and fitter may have to compete with the sub-personality that would rather sit at home, overeat and do no physical exercise. They are both parts of the same person but will have different aims and intentions. The part that wants to sit at home will experience the short-term payoffs of immediate comfort provided by food and inactivity, which reinforce the desire to do this. The part that wants to be healthier will need to be encouraged as the payoffs can be more long term.

Many schools of thought propose that where there are any sub-personalities the aim should be an integration of any and all. However, I wonder if a more powerful approach would be to understand and utilise various parts in different situations. That way a particular part that is useful for a given goal could be encouraged, strengthened and effectively used to pursue that goal. So rather than a homogenisation, a celebration of difference. Thus creating a mechanism of psychological teamwork.

Activity

Consider a goal or outcome that you want but have not yet achieved.

Rather than thinking that one part of you is good or superior to another take a little time to consider the following:

Which part of you (which sub-personality) really wants this goal or outcome?

For what purpose? Why is it important?

Which part of you (which sub-personality) is resisting?

For what purpose? Why is whatever this part wants instead important?

What qualities and strengths does each part have?

How can the part that wants the goal be strengthened while still honouring what the other part wants?

As part of my work I routinely use hypnosis, mindfulness, guided imagination and visualisations to assist clients to engage with and encourage their sub-personalities. It is often easier to work with someone else to do this type of exercise, but it is possible to do it on your own.

After considering the questions above perhaps take some time to not just think but also write your responses. You use a different part of your brain to write and many people believe this enhances the usefulness of the creative process. Then find a place and a time where you can relax, get comfortable but stay aware and alert. Otherwise you may just drift off to sleep.

Allow your imagination to create for you a way to symbolically envisage in any way that is appropriate to you the different parts or sub-personalities that are in conflict over this goal. There is no right way or wrong way of doing this. Any way you do it is perfect for you. In your mind's eye see these parts as separate to you, so that "you" become an objective observer of this guided daydream. With practice this will enable you to explore the symbolic experience of engaging with these sub-personalities. You will be able to discover how best to use their different qualities and power, rather than struggling or fighting or blaming one or the other. Raising your awareness in this way generates greater self-responsibility and enhances the quality of the relationship you have with yourself. In order to achieve your desired outcomes and fulfil your goals a healthy respect and deeper understanding of the various aspects of your sub-personalities is incredibly useful. All of the energy that you used to expend on struggling can be used to fulfil your potential. A good relationship with yourself is also reflected in the relationships you can enjoy with others.

As the objective observer, engage with each part and discover what they need to work together or at the very least to cease the conflict or struggle interfering with the attainment of the goal. Be respectful to each and grateful for their willingness to participate. At the conclusion of the exploration agree a plan of action that utilises the best of each.

The art of mentally rehearsing

A great way of creating your future history right now is to engage in a little bit of positive mental rehearsal. We often mentally rehearse up and coming situations. It is a natural activity for human beings. What is interesting though is that in an attempt to be prepared for all the things we do not want to happen, we mentally rehearse all the negatives. How about using the ability to mentally rehearse a situation that has not yet happened, but this time to put a more positive spin on the story?

It has been said that in neurological terms there is little difference between a real experience and one that is vividly imagined in detail. It is as if there is a part of us that thinks we have already actually done something if we vividly imagine it. And often when you have successfully done something once, it lays down a kind of blueprint in your mind that makes it easier next time.

In any way that is appropriate for you, take some time where you will not be distracted and relax your mind. One way of doing this is to practise the following "centring" exercise.

Centring Exercise

The centring exercise aims to bring about a union of the conscious and the unconscious that embodies harmony and balance. Use it to open, clear and change the flow of energy and raise awareness of sensory, mental, emotional and spiritual experience of being in the world in this moment. To develop a state of detached awareness, acceptance and integrity. Decide to be more compassionate and empathetic to self and others. This brief reflective exercise can enhance focus and concentration, and develop a greater sense of connecting to purpose and meaning.

Sit comfortably but alert, hands palms up on knees.

Imagine your body from the navel to the collarbone is like a container that you are filling with breath a 3rd at a time:

first you fill up the lower 3rd (the navel),
then the next 3rd (the ribs),
then all the way to the rim (the collarbones).

When you exhale imagine you are pouring out the air a little at a time. Start with a natural breath and eventually try to make the exhale last as long as the inhale.

Begin to develop awareness rather than being attached to any activity or content.

Notice who the "I" is that is watching / observing all this.

I am here in this room with my feet on the floor

I am here in this room with…

I am here in the room and…

I am here in my body but my body is not all that I am

I am thinking my thoughts but my thoughts are not me

I am engaged with my feelings but I am more than my feelings

I am

I am

I am

And I am more than all of this.

Set aside everything that is not relevant in this moment to this task… (Acknowledge and say I am setting aside X Y Z).

Set your intention (my intention right now is…).

Be at one with all that is useful in this moment.

Bring all this back to the now.

Mental Rehearsal

Then just allow pictures and sounds to emerge in your mind. Imagine that you are looking up at yourself as if looking at someone else. And see yourself performing whatever it is just the way you hope it will go. A best case scenario if you like. The more detailed and vivid you can make this imagined scene the better. Notice how the scene looks. Imagine in full Technicolor and moving images. Life size or perhaps even bigger and brighter. Hear any and all accompanying sounds. Listen to your own internal dialogue. What you are telling yourself?

Sometimes it can be useful to imagine someone else who does this really excellently and watch and listen to them. Including imagining what they say to themselves.

Now, if this is a mental movie, you are the director. So you can adjust, tweak and edit it until you are completely satisfied with the final version.

Then step into the main character. Whether it is you or someone else. Imagine actually doing what you watched. Get a sense of seeing through your eyes, hearing with your ears and feeling your emotions and the sensations associated with this experience.

If for whatever reason something does not feel quite right, then step out and take the observing movie director's role again. Once you have made any necessary further adjustments, step back in. You now have a perfect version that you can run in your mind, mentally rehearse whenever you want to in preparation.

If you want to you can take it a step further and add in some challenges so that you can mentally prepare handling any difficulties.

Six
It's not a mystery, actions have consequences.

I f you are in a relationship that is unfulfilling, you are not a victim; this is a consequence of your actions. If you are in a career that you hate this is a consequence of your previous decisions. If you are overweight you do not have a "weight problem", it is a consequence of your actions. I bet you could trace back and discover the actions that led to where you are now. When I say actions I also include inaction because even doing nothing is the action of failing to take action. Even refusing to make a decision is in fact deciding not to decide!

If you want to grow strawberries don't plant tomatoes. Don't blame the fruit because this is merely the outward result of what was planted. The seeds are where change needs to be made. Often we focus on the fruits rather than turning our attention to what was planted. Our inner world of thoughts and feelings creates our outer world of consequences. Just as the fruits are dictated by the seeds.

Once you have decided what you want it is then time to start working out how you get it. Decide on the destination then plan the route. Just as you have to decide what seeds to plant in order to get the desired fruit. Planning is essential. But planning alone is not enough. You then have to actually do what needs to be done to get what you want.

Failure has a structure. Success is not an accident. A saying I heard a while ago which I thought was so true was, "It's not that successful people know things that unsuccessful people don't know. It's that successful people are willing to do what unsuccessful people are not prepared to do".

The problem with the Jeremy Kyle generation... is that they want the privilege of rights without responsibility. Many avidly watch this daytime reality talk show where the host pokes and strokes, shouts and soothes in an attempt to "help" his guests with his own unique style of straight talking tough love. Of course, I suspect the programme is merely intended to make the rest of us who are watching, as opposed to appearing on the show, feel better about our lives. The guests often typify the 21st century desire for instant gratification without effort. Attitudes of "fix me", "do it for me", "it's not my fault".

If what you are doing isn't working - do something else. This statement is a great example of real common sense which is not always common practice. It is said that the definition of madness is to do the same thing over and over and expect a different result. But how often in everyday life do we do this? We indulge in habits of living. Like a fly trying to escape a hot conservatory, flying at the same closed window again and again and again. As if next time the window will miraculously disappear or at least be open. We may hit the same obstacle head on again and again in the vain hope or misguided expectation that it will crumble. Don't get me wrong, success usually requires at least an element of persistence. This is important. You can't do 10 sit ups and expect to have perfectly chiselled abs. If you leap up and look in the mirror you are likely to be disappointed. There is a need for consistency in taking effective action. Persistence at doing what works. Noticing feedback, monitoring the results you are getting, doing more of what gets you the results you want and less of what does not.

I remember I once had a client who was involved in the design of aircraft navigation equipment. He told me something that I had always thought was perhaps merely urban myth. He said that for much of the time they are in flight, aeroplanes are actually off their expected course.

However, the crew don't throw in the towel turn round and go home. This client told me that, "So long as you know where you have been and you are clear about where you are heading, then within reason wherever you are is fine providing you monitor the situation and consistently do what needs to be done to get to where you want to go." Now that, I thought, is a wonderful metaphor for life.

Think of an area of your life where you have an outcome that you have not yet achieved... and ask yourself honestly...

What have I been doing to get me where I am?

What do I need to do differently to get back on track to achieve my outcome?

Where do I need to focus my attention to make significant changes?

What do I need to do more of or less of?

What do I need to start doing or stop doing in order to get the results I want?

Responsibility vs. Blame

Many people do not like to accept the notion of consequences or personal responsibility. Instead they may feel more comfortable with the notion of blaming others. We exist in a time in history, at a stage of human evolution and in a culture where nothing apparently is our own fault. Where you could be forgiven for thinking that we are responsible for nothing. Our culture has developed into one of blame. Where many people actively seek to hold accountable someone or something else, outside of themselves for the conditions of their lives. To the ludicrous extent that if I eat nothing but fast food and as a result I get fat and sick I can blame the fast food company for creating, producing and selling me the stuff. Rather than have to take any responsibility for the consequences of my own decisions and actions, I can be absolved. It is consequences, both positive and negative, good and bad that create who we are, where we are and what we have right now. You are the sum total of everything that has gone before. Your life is the result of how you have lived up to this point. Let's get something straight here; I am not saying this as a judgment or criticism, it is merely an observation. Whatever has so far worked for you in life, where you have been successful, it is useful to note, acknowledge, celebrate and learn so you can replicate what works. Where you have not got the result you anticipated or wanted, consider the notion that there is no such thing as failure only feedback. Again acknowledge this, not to berate yourself but to learn from what has gone before in order to avoid repeating the same pitfalls.

So It's All My Fault?

Yes. In a way. And that is the good news! Good news? Yes it is, because if it wasn't your fault then you could, in the short term, sit back relieved and absolved of responsibility, shrug and say there is nothing I can do. However, in the long term this would be truly awful because it would mean you are helpless, hopeless and powerless to change things in your own life. If you accept responsibility then that might seem tough in the short term, however, in the long term it puts you in a wonderful position of power. Not power over other people but power to change and improve your life. You become literally empowered to do something to improve your lot in life.

Take A Look At The Results You Are Getting In Life.

What are your relationships like? For some people the answer to an unhappy relationship is to jump ship and find someone new. This is one solution. However, it can be a salutary experience to realise that what you thought would make you happy doesn't. It may be comforting to fool yourself into thinking that if your relationship isn't working it is all the fault of the other person. Relationships are not static things. They are dynamic processes which we engage in. Therefore rather than blaming the other person, it may be more useful to decide how the way you are relating to them needs to change in order to improve the quality of the relationship.

If you just change to someone new without addressing the underlying cause of the problems, it can lead to "different cast / same script" syndrome. You can change the players involved but if you continue to do the same things you are likely to get the same eventual result. If you have problems with various people in different areas of your life then it might be useful to take a look to see what is the common denominator? The answer is, you.

Sometimes we mistake short term pleasure for long term satisfaction. In the short term it may be easier and more pleasurable to lie on the sofa and eat doughnuts, but in the long term what pain will that lead to?

In the short term it may be more exciting to skip to a new partner but in the long term if you can't make a relationship work through good times and bad, then you are unlikely to experience the deep satisfaction that accompanies a lasting partnership. We may attempt to avoid any discomfort in the misguided idea that this is what brings happiness. We want quick and easy fixes, seek short term pleasure and fool ourselves that there are no negative consequences. Instead of moaning about how hard it is, or looking for the quick and easy fix, just get on with doing what needs to be done and acknowledge that if it was easy then anyone would do it. And you are not just anyone.

The road to mastery is persistence and practice. In any endeavour the requirement for success involves the discipline to keep on doing what needs to be done. The decisions you make when things get tough determine your character and long term success. Anyone can have a positive attitude when life is easy.

Physically, if you are fat (or unhealthy or unfit) it is likely to be the consequence of your actions (or inaction). The lifestyle choices, unhealthy habits and the impact on the body of high fat processed foods and not enough exercise. I am not an advocate of the idea that every illness you experience is created by some deed or thought. Sometimes stuff does just happen. Chemical reactions. Predispositions of cells. Genetic disposition. However, there is always something that you can be in control of. As Maya Angelou said, "Just because you are in pain, doesn't mean you have to be one."

We Create Our Own Reality.

As Henry Ford said, "Whether you think you can or whether you think you can't, you're probably right."

The second of "Clarke's Three Laws" of prediction formulated by the British writer and scientist Arthur C. Clarke states that: "The only way of discovering the limits of the possible is to venture a little way past them into the impossible."

The truth is that in life we often do not know exactly what is possible until we actually do it. Often people limit what they believe is possible due to a lack of confidence. As a result I genuinely believe that we do create our own reality.

I am not talking from an existential or even a metaphysical perspective, but more literally than that. Now, I am in no way suggesting that we are to "blame" for all of the circumstances of our lives. We cannot always control what happens to us. However, we can control what we choose to focus on in any given situation.

"We see the world not how it is but how we are" is a wonderful quote which has been used by many people so I do not claim to know the original source of it. We literally understand the world around us through the veil of who we are. The brilliant news is that this can and does change. As we evolve via knowledge gained though experience, providing we don't try too hard to keep things the same, providing we embrace ambiguity and uncertainty so that we can benefit from the range of experience that is available to us. Children encounter the world from a "know nothing" state. If as adults we could adopt this we would be able to truly expand our knowledge without preconceived ideas. We could learn rather than seeking merely to confirm what we think we already know.

Carl Jung the psychologist said that all perception is projection. Meaning that in order to recognise something in others we have to have it within our own self. We fool ourselves into thinking that we experience the world, reality and events but actually we are responding to our own interpretations, our own thoughts and feelings about what is happening. I think the saying, "it is all in your head" is really funny because where else can anything be? The only place you can exist is in your own head, in your own mind.

Just in case you are intrigued about the other two here are all 3 of "Clarke's Laws"

*1. When a distinguished but elderly scientist states that something is **possible**, he is almost certainly right. When he states that something is **impossible,** he is very probably wrong.*

2. The only way of discovering the limits of the possible is to venture a little way past them into the impossible

3. Any sufficiently advanced technology is indistinguishable from magic.

Seven
Is fear keeping you stuck?

Okay, so deep down you know what you really want. Whether that's in terms of what you want from a relationship, or what you would really like to do as a career, or something else. So if you know what you want, what's holding you back? What's preventing you from getting on with doing what needs to be done, in order to achieve what you REALLY want? The answer is likely to come down to some kind of FEAR. Now, although not a pleasant feeling, fear is not a bad thing. Fear is in fact a necessary element of the human survival instinct. Without it the human race would have become extinct a long time ago. However, many of the things that we are afraid of in the 21st century are really nowhere near as bad as our imaginations make them out to be. We may fear doing the wrong thing, making the wrong decision, losing something that we already have so that our position gets worse instead of better. We may fear how we will appear to others and what they will think of us. The list of 'what if' questions can seem endless. It's as if the thinking part of us wants to come up with answers for every possible consequence so that the emotional part of us feels okay. The truth is, it's impossible to really know the extent of an outcome prior to taking action. *Foresight is never perfect. Only hindsight can be 20/20.*

5 Simple Questions

When I work with my coaching or NLP clients who want to make a change but are holding back, I get them to consider 5 key questions:

1. What is the worst that could happen?

Now this may seem a bit on the negative side, however, considering what the worst possible outcome of some decision or action is, in a rational way can be really useful. Although we may be consumed with anxiety we often avoid or skirt around actually thinking this through.

Once you have fully considered and described the worst possible outcome, the "what if it all goes wrong" scenario, you are then ready to consider the next question.

2. What could you or would you do if this did happen? Very often just realising that you would cope and get through it is very liberating.

Then consider:

3. **What is the very best that could happen?** Again, think about and describe this in as much detail as you can. This can begin the shift from feeling afraid about what might go wrong, to feeling excited about what could go right.

4. **What if you do nothing and stay exactly the same as you are now?** Although, of course, in reality this is not possible. Even though some people fear change, change is inevitable. Improvement is optional.

Having considered all this you are in a much better position to decide:

5. **On balance, is what it's possible to gain worth the risk?**

The Secret of "NTNK"

While my son was learning to surf in Bali, he had a terrifying experience. Out of nowhere he was hit by a big freak wave. The power of it knocked him off the board. Suddenly he was engulfed in a huge wall of roaring water which dragged him down faster and deeper than he had ever been. Within a second it was like being inside a giant washing machine. The force of the wave spun him round and round and dragged him further down. It felt like an age before finally he broke free. Battered, bruised, terrified and disorientated he literally felt as if he was in a fight for his life. He had no idea which way was up. Still somehow holding his breath he began to swim in the direction of what he hoped was the surface. It was little more than sheer guesswork.

Just as he felt as if his lungs would burst he emerged coughing and spluttering from the depths to the surface. The wave had dragged him some distance out to sea, so the swim back to shore was exhausting. Finally he dragged himself up the beach to where the archetypal laid-back instructors were sunbathing.

He recounted every detail of the nightmarish experience as they listened attentively.

'Oh yeah, that happens on this stretch of coast sometimes,' one of the instructors casually remarked.

'Why didn't you warn me?'

'Because, truth is, if it's going to happen no one can prepare you for it. Plus if we had told you it was a possibility, you wouldn't have gone in.'

'No, too right I wouldn't.'

'And you wouldn't have learned that even though it was really tough, you could handle it.'

Somewhat reluctantly he had to agree they had a point.

'Will it be okay next time?' he asked, hoping for some reassurance.

With a wry smile the instructor replied, 'NTNK... never try never know.'

Eight
The pitfalls of mind-reading

T he truth is that it is not possible to know what someone else is thinking even though lots of people spend lots of time and energy trying to mind-read, or expecting others to be able to read their minds. If we know someone really well we may be able to predict with some accuracy what makes them tick and how they are likely to respond in certain situations. This level of accurate prediction can make us falsely believe that we are good at reading people. We can become even more convinced we know what others think. Each correct prediction, either due to sheer luck, or perhaps an intelligent guess based on previous experience, strengthens the erroneous belief that it is possible to know the thoughts of another.

When we mind–read, a pitfall is that we are in fact telling ourselves a story. And the danger of this is that we behave in accordance with that story. We may believe that we know how someone thinks and based on this we tell ourselves a story created around how we think the other person is going to react. If it does not work out the way we expect and the meanings etc. we attributed to their actions and words based on our mind-read turn out to be inaccurate we get upset. We are not in fact upset by the other person, although this might be what we say. We have in fact upset ourselves by the story we created in our own mind based on mind-reading. It is almost as if we view the world in flat 2D monochrome, when in fact it is 3D and glorious Technicolor. There exist connections and inter-connections beyond our wildest imaginings. Rather than being open and seeing and experiencing what is actually there, we get lost in our own fantasy story of what we think should or ought to be there. What might happen if you played with the idea that "nothing means anything, until or unless we decide that it does"? What would happen if every time you thought you knew what something meant that you asked, "What else could this mean?" "What else could be going on?" "What might be an alternative story from the obvious that I could tell myself?" "What might someone else say about this from their perspective?" It is not that we are wrong or being untruthful. It is just that we see things how we see them and we do not know what we do not know, until we do. Think about the disparities between eyewitness statements or the reminiscence of family members over past events. If you look for possible alternatives to your automatic responses to things, people and situations this will broaden your perspective.

Henry Ford said, 'Whether you think you can or whether you think you can't, you are probably right.' We act as if our beliefs are facts. When in reality beliefs are strongly held opinions. Beliefs are thoughts. Thoughts affect feelings. Feelings affect behaviour, which affects results. The results we get in turn support our beliefs. Either consciously or unconsciously we seek evidence that supports what we believe. We ignore or dismiss as fluke what doesn't fit what we expect. Considering beliefs in this way negates the necessity to decide if something is right or wrong, true or false. Instead you can look to see if a belief is useful or helpful to you in a particular context. There are really only two types of belief. Those that are useful and empower us and those that are not useful and somehow limit us. If beliefs are not facts you can decide to keep only those useful ones that empower you. Wherever the others came from you can decide to ditch them. What results might you get if you decided to just play with the idea of challenging your limiting beliefs? What if you believed you could? What would you then be free to do? What might you accomplish?

Nine
Positive attitude rather than positive thinking

P ositive thinking is not realistic and can be delusional… pretending that everything is wonderful when it is not prevents you from doing what needs to be done, facing up to how things are and identifying how to get from where you are to where you want to be. We can't influence the cards we are dealt, only how we play our hand. Negative thinking is unrealistic too because just as nothing is all good, nothing is all bad either. Honest thinking, that is not pretending things are better than they are, but certainly not pretending that they are worse than they actually are either can lead to a resilience. A certain knowledge that whatever happens, you will deal with it.

Inspiring Examples of a Positive Attitude

The following are, in my opinion, two great examples of people who have retained a positive attitude even when faced with adversity. **Randy Pausch** was an American professor at Carnegie Mellon University. He became a worldwide internet sensation when his "last lecture" was featured on

YouTube. Pausch discovered that he had pancreatic cancer in September 2007 and was told it was terminal. He died in July 2008 leaving a wife and three young children. **Nick Vujicic** was born in 1982 in Melbourne, Australia. Without any medical explanation or warning, he came into the world with neither arms nor legs. Having had an uneventful pregnancy and no family history to expect this condition, imagine the shock his parents, Nurse Dushka Vujicic, and her husband Pastor Borris Vujicic, felt when they saw their first-born, brand new baby boy. A limbless child was not what had been expected. How would their son live a normal happy life? What could he ever do or become when living with what the world would see as such a massive disability? Little did they know that one day he would inspire and motivate people from all walks of life, touching lives all over the world.

We are all part of the human race, but we do not all start from the same place or run at the same pace. Some people have lots of advantages; for example, loving supportive families, financial security, physical or intellectual prowess. Our life chances and opportunities may well be impacted by when and where we happen to be born. However, these things do not ultimately define you as a human being. That is not unless you decide that they do. An honest evaluation of where you are starting from and where you want to get to, together with an evaluation of what needs to be done and whether you are in fact prepared to do what needs to be done to get where you say you want to be… are all important.

No one can do it for you. No one can want it for you. Only you can do it for yourself. Often the solution to our problems, or at least the thing that would be very helpful, is if other people changed. You can't change anyone else in the world except yourself. Even if it seems as if our lives would be so much better if others were different. Take a long hard honest look at yourself and make some choices about where you are going to focus your energy.

Consider the idea that we may not always be masters of our own destiny; however, we do create our own reality. Human beings experience the world via five senses; that is, we can touch, taste, smell, see and hear. Unless there is a sensory impairment, we all use all of these senses. We will have certain unconscious preferences. And this will impact on where we focus our attention and what we notice. The brain combines the input of our two eyes into a single three-dimensional image. Even though the image on the retina is upside down because of the focusing action of the lens, the brain compensates and provides a right side up perception.

The spectrum of light to which the human eye is sensitive varies from the red to the violet. Lower electromagnetic frequencies (infrared) and higher frequencies (ultraviolet) cannot be detected. The human eye is not sensitive to the polarisation of light, i.e. light that oscillates on a specific plane. The average person with normal hearing experiences between 20Hz on the low side and approximately 20,000Hz on the high side. Sound above or below this is simply outside of the audible range of human hearing. So in a sense, even this first access to the external world is filtered. We experience only a thin slice of what we perceive as "external reality" in comparison to what is potentially there. Then inside of our own minds we have another set of personal filters which are made up of our experiences, memories and various preferences in terms of how we extract and sort information from the input from the world. These personal filters create our internal representations. That is, we literally re-present the external world inside our own minds. Just as a map is only a representation of the actual terrain surveyed, just as a meal is just a representation of the meals on offer, so our internal representations are only a representation of the external world.

However, we work on the assumption that our internal representations ARE the same as external reality. We understand things largely by reference to what we already know. Therefore we edit the input based on previous experiences and expectations. These processes are largely unconscious rather than premeditated.

We do not know what we do not know until we do. Nothing means anything until we decide it does. Our experience of objective reality is probably a lot more subjective that we perhaps thought. Two good examples of this are: 1. When you try to reminisce with family or friends and end up with very different versions of seemingly the same experience. 2. Eyewitness statements of the same scene. While not purposely misleading or untrue, are simply good examples of how what you notice about a situation or event will largely be determined by what you focus on, where you place your attention and what you are expecting.

It is widely accepted that women have a better peripheral ability. This supposedly is due to evolution where females had to be able to scan the horizon in order to detect danger well enough in advance to protect the young. Whereas men are more focused on one target, either to hunt and kill or protect the tribe from threat. Maybe this explains why your man cannot see what is in front of him as he stares in the fridge or cupboard telling you that whatever it is you said was there, isn't. And how when you point it out he thinks it is some kind of feminine trickery.

We create our own reality by projecting what is within ourselves onto the world and other people. By acting as if our beliefs are facts rather than strongly held opinions. By the meanings that we attribute to the hand we are dealt. By the way we physiologically and psychologically filter the world and external events.

Knowledge of this gives us choice and flexibility so that never again can you say, that is just the way that it is. That it is simply a fact of reality. Because it is, after all, subjective. If there are many more ways to literally see and interpret everything, then are you focusing on the most helpful, useful and beneficial ways of doing this? Forget what it right or wrong, true of false. Is the way you are creating your world the most helpful for you in terms of what you want and the life you want to lead?

Ten
Are you caught between "what if?" and "if only?"

> "There are only two days in the year that nothing can be done.
>
> One is called yesterday and the other is tomorrow"
>
> **Dalai Lama**

What if… is about the future. If only… is about the past. Recalling, imagining and evaluating both can be useful. However, if you spend too much time mentally and emotionally in either the past or the future, what you miss out on is the present. Encouraging yourself to adopt a mindset of keeping present moment awareness, rather than slipping into the illusion of past or future, neither of which actually exists in the present except in your own mind, is an essential element to mastering your mind.

Just stop for a moment and consider, what is actually going on in this immediate present moment? What can you actually see, hear, taste, smell, and feel?

What are the quality and content of your thoughts right now?

If you were to just sit for a moment where would your thoughts wander?

Could you remain in this present moment without thinking of what you have to do in the near or distant future, or what you have already done or what has already happened in the past?

In this present moment what problems do you actually have? In reality what problems are you experiencing right now? I don't mean what is coming up or what you're currently worried about. I mean in this moment, if this was all there is, what problems, difficulties or challenges do you actually have right now?

You may find that the negatives are all attached either to the past, to what has already happened... the "if onlys". Or to the future, dreading and worrying about what is to come, the "what if's". "What if" thoughts are about what could or might happen in the future. This type of thinking often creates feelings of anxiety which, because they are experienced in the present moment, are confused with feeling bad about the present moment. So even though there may be nothing actually happening in the present moment to be anxious about, the negative effects of what-if-ing impacts the present even though it is concern about the future, about what is yet to come, that creates these negative thoughts.

"If only's" are thoughts about the past, about what did or did not happen the way you would have preferred. "If only's" are re-runs of events, or in some cases a fantasy, about what should or should not have occurred. These "if only" thoughts create a negativity that is mistaken as belonging to the present. Both "what if's" and "if only's" are insidious illusions. Tricks of your thinking. If they go unchallenged it is seductive to believe that as if by worrying or engaging in negative thinking somehow you will be able to prevent future problems or somehow edit the past. This is blatantly not the case.

If you do engage in what-if-ing or if–only-ing… do you imagine that the future will perhaps be better than the present? In effect do you play the "I'll be happy when" game?

Or if you are a more traditional pessimist you probably make yourself suitably miserable by expecting things to deteriorate even further. "Things are, of course, bad now, but they're going downhill fast so the future will be even worse!" Are you a creative negative thinker who can recall the past in some rosy glow of nostalgia as better than now?

Those were the best days of my life and now they are a very long time ago. Or do you allow your imagination free rein to remember the past as even worse than it actually was? After all, if it was really that awful how did you survive it to live until now?

Memory is reconstructive rather than accurately reproductive. That is, by the very act of remembering we embellish our past even if we don't consciously mean to. A good example of this is when people reminisce. How often do people agree when they recall a shared experience? How often do people recall exactly the same details from a shared event?

All of our experiences happen in the present moment, we then file them away and augment them as we remember. This is not a conscious decision to be somehow untruthful. It just happens. Think about it for a moment. How many of your memories are just okay, just average? That is, as it was, no better no worse?

The simple truth is that you have created the present you have via processes of cause and effect. Every decision you have made, every decision you have avoided, every action you have taken, every action you have avoided taking, these have all contributed to who you are and where you are and what you have right now. The circumstances of your life are not what determine whether or not you are happy, positive, successful or fulfilled. You may believe that it is the quality of your relationships, or how much or how little money you have, or what your family background is. However, if that was the truth, all rich people would be happy and all poor people miserable. Everyone who is loved would be well adjusted and positive. Those with financially and/or emotionally secure backgrounds would, without fail, be happy. And vice versa. And even a glimpse in the direction of one of the many magazines dedicated to the lifestyles of the rich and famous confirms that this is not the case.

It is not even knowledge or good education that guarantees an ability to think positively. In some cases ignorance is bliss. When you don't know what you don't know it can be wonderfully liberating. It is true, however, that ignorance and lack of education can also be the source of misery. When you don't know what you don't know it can be difficult to identify and then locate the resources you require. Like wanting to go on holiday but having no concept of what different locations have to offer. In order to make an informed choice it can be useful to be shown a selection of brochures. On the other hand if the only place you ever went on holiday was Clacton and you had a great time, going somewhere more exotic would not necessarily enhance your level of enjoyment, even if it did enrich your experience base.

The present moment is all that truly exists because the past is over and the future has not yet happened. So one simple way to master your mind and improve your emotional experience straight away is to just decide to start to be happier right now in this the present moment. Believing that the future will be better, is not an excuse to leave it to that future you, who will somehow be more motivated, more intelligent or more self-disciplined. This is not an excuse to be inactive and leave the future in the hands of fate. The message is not to merely enjoy the present moment with pure unabashed hedonism. But to be happier and think more positively, to enjoy fully and appreciate to the maximum this present moment; with whatever is, or is not happening right now. While at the same time to strive, to plan and to take the necessary actions to achieve more for the future.

If it is the past that appears to be the problem, if on some level you have told yourself (and maybe anyone else who cared to listen) that any negative conditions in your present life are somehow the result of what has already happened to you, you are in serious danger of confusing history with destiny. The truth is that the only way your future is dictated by your past is if you decide that it is.

Think about this... the present you are living right now, is the future you once looked forward to. And today is tomorrow's yesterday.

ACTIVITY: bring your awareness back to the present moment. To the reality of where you are and what you are doing right now. Decide to create some distance from the future and the past and simply experience the here and now for what it is. No more, no less. No better but certainly no worse than it actually is. Notice whenever your thinking leaps forward to imagine an anxiety provoking future or slips back to assess the past in some negative way and make a decision to focus only on the present and what is actually occurring right now.

21st century epidemic of depression. I want to state categorically that what follows are merely my individual ponderings, opinions, beliefs and questions about the 21st century epidemic of depression. I am not, however, in any way implying that I do not think this horrible illness is not 'real'. I, for one, have personal experience of how very real depression is. Even in the 21st century there is real stigma and misunderstanding of mental health issues. As I write this, news that comedian and actor Robin Williams took his own life after experiencing many years of addiction and depression has brought the subject of mental health to the world's attention, at least for a day or so! Although it has become a talking point, the level of ignorance is almost unbelievable. People say, but he was talented, rich, successful, famous, loved and admired, what did he have to be depressed about? As if depression is some kind of lifestyle choice.

The scars and the on-going life threatening symptoms of mental illness may be mostly invisible to the naked eye, and "sufferers" certainly do not make great "poster campaign" victims. In fact we are often treated as if our illness is somehow our own responsibility. As if it is our fault and we should be able to snap out of it, or think more positive, happy thoughts.

The origins or causes of this horrible illness are unclear: is it lifestyle, life experience, genetics, or a complex mix of all these casual elements? I can say with some certainty that personally I think I have experienced depression my whole life. Although my parents were loving and tried to help support me, doing the very best with what they knew, I was a deeply troubled and unhappy child. I can honestly say that while I never experienced any real trauma or abuse in my formative years, still I was ill. I was first prescribed dosulepin for major depressive disorder when I was just 14. By which time my thoughts, behaviour and lifestyle had already become reckless and self-punishing. As a result perhaps of the medication, I did not commit suicide but can honestly say that other than that it did not feel as if it helped much. I continued to be a depressed teenager and than a depressed young person. I underwent counselling but it wasn't until I was given my first prescription for Prozac in my 30s that I can honestly say I remember thinking for the very first time in my life… this must be what it feels like to be normal.

I do not hold with the notion that I "battle", "struggle" or am a "victim" of this condition. Instead I accept, I acknowledge and perhaps even embrace it as an integral part of me, of who I am.

As my life experience progressed I think that my interest and drive to study therapy and become a people-helper was at least in part due to the fact that I was always seeking my own personal cure. Although, so far, I have to say that I have not found it, along the way I have learned so much and acquired so much knowledge and expertise that I am blessed to have helped many other people fulfil their potential. Plus I think I have (mostly) broken the terrible legacy of depression passing down my family line. And where this has not been possible I have assisted those afflicted to get effective help. I have learned how to mostly, most of the time, manage my condition and my life so that life is sweet and I love what I do, love what I have and who I am and experience the best life I can… at least most of the time. In the past I was secretive about my condition because as a therapist and trainer of therapists I felt embarrassed, ashamed even, as if I was a fraud. If I could not heal myself what business did I have offering help to others? Gradually I realised that in the process of seeking to help myself I acquired the skills to help many, many, other people. Plus I use what I know on a daily basis to better manage my own condition.

Now, I have heard conspiracy theorists suggest the epidemic of depression is due to the billions of pounds it makes for pharmaceutical companies in revenue for anti-depressant medications. And maybe it is true that for some time-poor GPs it is easier to write a prescription than have a conversation that may spill over the allotted appointment time. Therapy is expensive and can be a bit of a lottery in terms of whether it turns out to be a good investment or not. I believe that some types of therapy are at best ineffective and at worst in danger of re-traumatising people. Therapy, despite the rise in popularity for Cognitive Behavioural Therapy (CBT), is not a one-size-fits-all cure. The relationship between therapist and client, it has been said, can be more a significant determinant of a successful outcome than the therapeutic orientation of the therapist. What is not in doubt, to me at least, is that many people feel unable to reveal their deepest angst even to family or friends. And certainly not to work colleagues. Depression is still regarded by some as a weakness of character. I have had private clients who could have accessed therapy at no charge to themselves through their employers, but chose not to for fear that it might jeopardise future career prospects.

A Spiritual Crisis?

Personally I do wonder if partly, for some people at least, depression is caused by, or exacerbated by, a widespread spiritual crisis. For many there appears to be a sad disconnection from who we are and why we are. Some turn to radical religions that merely emphasise the differences between people and spread fear and tribalism. Some look towards the consumer-driven spirituality without substance, of unicorns and dolphins. In the midst of crowded cities, people experience isolation and alienation and feelings of inadequacy fuelled at least in part by the emphasis on consumerism and hedonism. Life can appear meaningless and we can feel powerless if we are unable to be, do or have it all and live a truly "awesome" life. We are bombarded by hollow ideals of fame and fortune or of living meaningful lives filled with a sincere passion for what we do. For many, the mundane reality of life can be less inspiring. Many great philosophers and psychologists have attempted to understand and explain the human condition and our need to personally evolve and fulfil our potential. And in recent times there has been acknowledgement of the importance of finding or creating some meaning and purpose in life. I do not pretend to have the answers. But I think the questions are interesting.

A few conclusions on mastering your mind:

"If you think education is expensive, try ignorance."

Mastering you mind is about opening up to alternative options. You don't know what you don't know, until you do. It is useful to develop the awareness that your mind is at the same time both your most valuable ally and potentially your most dangerous opponent. Mastering your mind is the art of realising that your outer world is at least in part the creation of your inner world. This is empowering but for some people a little scary. In order to expand your mind it is useful to be able to distinguish between information and opinion. One way to do this effectively is through education. It doesn't have to be formal education, although the rigour and discipline of academic study is a good grounding discipline in being able to make informed decisions. The autodidact, the self-taught person can be just as discerning. An education is valuable. Knowledge is power as they say. What you learn becomes a part of you. It can help explain why you are the way you are and who you are and help shape who you choose to become. It almost does not even matter what you decide to learn as long as you learn something. Learn as much as you can about what you want to and you become a specialist. Or learn in a shallow yet wide way so that you know a little about a lot of things. While you will never know everything there is to know, you can know what you know and also know that it is okay to keep learning. To keep expanding, growing and evolving.

Unlearning can also be a truly amazing aspect of mastering your mind. Unlearning the things you thought to be true, that restricted or limited you, perhaps the things you believed at one time were irrefutable facts only to discover they were in fact no more than opinions that had been passed on to you. This kind of unlearning can be truly liberating. It is impossible for anyone to learn what they think they already know. The ability to discern facts from opinion is becoming more and more of a challenge in the 21st century. Just because we see something, read something, are exposed to something does not mean it is necessarily true. Mastering your mind also involves developing your own intuition. After all, even irrefutable facts which are impossible to deny or disprove, incontrovertible reality, is confined to what is currently known and understood. Imagine trying to tell someone about the internet or explain Wi-Fi, back in 1970.

So continue to question and expand and test your knowledge and understanding gained through experience. Develop your capacity to reflect on your experience and appreciate that personal subjective experience is important but not all that there is to know. Keep an open mind.

Befriend your Body

Denise Collins

One

D o you need to lose weight?

Are you unhappy with your body?

Would you like to reverse the signs of aging?

Have you ever avoided doing something because of being unhappy about the the way you look?

What is the next big thing? What is the real deal?

It's not fat loss methods or fitness programmes or cosmetic procedures. I believe it is helping people to experience true body esteem. No nonsense, cut the bullshit misinformation, dump the latest fad diet, miracle potion crap and get educated. This is not about giving up, giving in or denial. This is a real process for real people that brings about positive personal improvement and even life transformation. The truth is that multi-billion pound and dollar industries are created and dependent on you being unhappy with who you are. The ideal image of what your physical appearance should be is, for some people, of such significance that it dominates every aspect of life. At the very least the perception of what we should aspire to look like has an insidious impact on the vast majority of us.

The real problem isn't weight management or even health issues. It is the culture of self-loathing that pervades the 21st century developed first world. It seems as if issues of size, shape, weight, age and aesthetics dominate our perception of not only how physically attractive we are considered but how successful or even worthy we are as human beings. Women have been judged like this for a long time, but now increasingly men are too.

Two

I magine that you are given something to take care of that is totally unique. It is quite literally one of a kind. And so once it is gone it is gone. There are similar models out there but this one is unique. It is both fragile and at the same time very robust. Not only is it unique, but it is also serviceable and practical too. It operates in complex ways that are wonderfully, amazingly mind-blowing. It is a piece of design capable of performing a multitude of life sustaining functions simultaneously. If it gets broken, damaged or neglected it is likely not to perform to its optimum.

How would you feel about being entrusted with such a rare and fascinating commodity?

What value do you think you might place upon this rare and precious thing?

Compare this to how you think and behave towards your own body.

I decided to call this system master your mind BEFRIEND your body because an issue for many people in the 21ˢᵗ century is that they actually hate their bodies. The discontent goes way beyond a simple dislike or non-acceptance of how they are physically. It spills over into a dangerous degree of self-revulsion. "My body is mine but it is not I". It is yours; it is the only one you have. It is precious and unique. But it is not all that you are. The comparisons we are encouraged to make between ourselves and those impossibly perfect images of gorgeous looking celebrities and beautiful icons fosters the notion of total non-acceptance of everyday imperfections. These can become regarded as totally intolerable rather than normal, natural and what makes you irreplaceable. An unhealthy contradiction as far as I am concerned, is just how many people attempt to address issues of health and wellbeing from a starting place of self-loathing. This is frankly quite senseless. Acceptance does not have to equate with giving up or condoning what is wrong. Acceptance could be thought of in the following way:

I Am A Carthorse.

If I am a carthorse no amount of attention to improving my nutrition, no amount of time spent in a gym or adhering to particular diets or exercise regimes will transform me into a racehorse. To try to achieve the impossible would be to doom myself to the disappointment of inevitable failure. And the rejection of who and what I am as defective rather than distinctive.

However, if I celebrate who and what I am, then I can focus all my attention and energy on taking the best care of myself, ensuring I am healthy and becoming the very best version of myself that is possible. Instead of trying in vain to be something I am never going to be (a racehorse) I can get on with enjoying the process of becoming the best me I can possibly be (a truly fabulous carthorse!)

Three
Why befriend your body?

Quite simply because it is the only one you have. It is yours but it is not all that you are. What might happen if you decided to love your body for all its individual imperfections and for the wonderfully perfect example of an everyday miracle that it is? What might happen if you chose to befriend it? Make the most of it? Enjoy it? And stop blaming it or hating it for the shape it is in. Truth is that if you are alive then essentially there is more right with your body than wrong with it. If you loathe your body you are unlikely to take care of it or make the most of it. To befriend your body is to counter the general 21st century obsession with dissatisfaction with physical appearance. The idea that we must all strive to be forever young, perfect, beautiful bodies. Beauty is not in the *Botox* because beauty is in fact a feeling. It is an experience.

Here are 3 ideas for beginning to befriend your body:

- Listen to the way you talk about your body to yourself and others. Create some positive affirmations based on acceptance and begin to repeat these to yourself on a daily basis
- Try seeing yourself through the eyes of someone who truly loves you
- Make a decision to notice and appreciate the many different ways that people can be beautiful

We are accustomed to being told what is beautiful, however, we can be fooled into forgetting that this actually changes (often very rapidly with fashions) and is influenced by the media, our culture, and the period in history in which we live. The body you have is the only one you've got. So it might be a good idea to befriend it rather than treating it like the enemy! How might it alter things if you thought of your body as the vehicle for your being?

Take a little time right now to consider your physical body. Perhaps go and take a good look at yourself in a mirror. What are your automatic reactions to what you see? How do you feel about your body? Are you content with it or dissatisfied? Do you focus on what you like or what you regard as faults? Do you consider that you are too fat, too thin, too short, too tall, too old, too young, too hairy, too bald or just about right? How do you take care of yourself? Are you fit or unhealthy? What words would you use to describe your body? How does your body feel on the inside? Is your body working effectively? What bodily sensations are you aware of? Do you have pain or discomfort? A lot has been said and written about the **impact of the media** on influencing our thoughts about body image and what constitutes physical standards of beauty. And sure enough there is evidence in all those re-touched, modified photographic images showing beautiful young women with impossibly long slender limbs, perfectly clear skin and defined contours. All those stick-thin prepubescent catwalk models and stunning performers. The cult of celebrity elevates certain people to fame and fortune just for looking a certain way. Although an emphasis is placed on the stressful impact this has on the young and impressionable, it is not restricted to them. There is increasing pressure on all people; male, female, young and older to conform to what is regarded as acceptable physical characteristics, shape, size and standardised notions of beauty. The reality is that fashions and fads around beauty are not a 21st century or even a new phenomenon. Throughout history and across all cultures, those people fortunate enough to be elevated from the daily grind of merely trying to survive have always been influenced by what is considered beautiful or attractive at a particular time in a certain place.

Fear of failure. Fear of rejection. I believe that many of the insecurities that abound about our physical bodies are merely indications of feelings of deeper insecurity, of somehow not being considered "good enough". Issues of confidence, our self-image and self-esteem are fused with ideas of what makes us acceptable. Get it wrong and there is the risk of failure. Get it wrong and you risk feeling unlovable and the resulting fear of rejection.

Perhaps the time has come for a new paradigm. Maybe it is time for a new movement towards genuine acceptance. Not pretending to tolerate that which we actually find intolerable. Not pretending to be happy with being unhealthy. Not deluding ourselves into a false self-approval because we simply cannot be bothered to take action to change what it is within our control to improve. But a self-acceptance of our unique individuality rather than a stream of self-criticism for being distinctive. True acceptance involves doing the best you can with what you have, rather than bemoaning the fact that you may never be considered super model material. Value your body enough to work on improving what you can. While lovingly accepting what can't be changed. And to borrow from the serenity prayer, having the wisdom to know the difference between these two.

Four
Your body and multi-billion pound industries.

The trend towards dissatisfaction with "ordinary" physical bodies has spawned a plethora of multi-billion pound industries. There is the diet industry, the fitness industry, the cosmetic surgery industry. There are non-surgical treatments, beauty salons, anti-aging serums and creams, spas and chains of gyms. If the main motive of any industry is to make a profit what is the relationship between what we think and how we feel about our bodies and these industries?

We are encouraged, some might say brainwashed, to be dissatisfied with our physical appearance and then sold stuff to correct the perceived shortcomings and imperfections. In spite of any real success we may have achieved in life, it seems as if we are solely judged or judge ourselves simply on how thin or toned we are or how youthful we look. Even intelligent people seem to adhere to the notion that if you are thin/buff and/or look young then your life as a direct consequence will be perfect. We are bombarded by explicit and implicit messages which imply that in order to have a happy, satisfying life you need to be young and fit-looking.

Befriend your body is about jumping off the treadmill (pardon the pun) of self-loathing because you are not how you think you ought to be physically. There is nothing wrong with healthy, happy body aspiration. However, the reality is more often that aspirations for a "better" body have their roots firmly in loathing and undermining the body you currently have. There have been various studies about how body image anxiety prevents people from participating in activities or taking advantage of opportunities. This is tragic. Human beings come in a widely diverse variety of models. We come in different combinations of colour, size and shape. If your focus is primarily on how you think you look while making negative comparison with how you think you should look, this occupies way too much headspace. This kind of obsessing about physical acceptability and attractiveness, based on external perceptions of what constitutes the ideal weight, shape, fitness levels, age and definition of beauty, is energy consuming. It prevents sincere, genuine relationships and the participation in real, present moment awareness.

Without realising it is happening we internalise standards of what constitutes physical attractiveness.

It is interesting to consider that the standard version of physical attractiveness is actually unattainable for the majority of the population. We are encouraged to pursue an ideal that we are unlikely ever to achieve. What does this do for our sense of individual self-esteem?

Although for a long time older men have been prized more highly than older women (older men are often portrayed as experienced, wise and therefore attractive, while older women are seen as unattractive and asexual), staying young-looking is becoming more and more important for both sexes. Men too it seems are now feeling the pressure to stay younger looking. There are an increasing number of products aimed exclusively at men, from hair dye to moisturiser and fitness magazines promising the secret to attaining that elusive six pack. The natural signs of aging are perceived as negative.

We are brainwashed into believing that to be loveable and successful we must banish those wrinkles and grey hair. Beauty is associated with youth. But none of us can turn the clock back so again we are being sold a version of youthful) beauty that is unattainable due to the natural process of aging. Even the wealthy that have access to the very best cosmetic surgeons can hold back time for only so long. Eventually they end up looking like a parody, a caricature of their younger self.

Befriending your body is not about giving up or giving in or letting yourself go. It is about discovering your own inherent values which is independent of your physical exterior. It is about living an authentic existence with who you are, in the body you have, so that you can be the best version of yourself according to what is right for you rather than what is right for the industries that regard you as merely a way of increasing their revenue.

When you are happier, this literally equates to being healthier. Life is about balance between mind and body, between physical, mental emotional wellbeing. If you take weight loss as an example, there are obvious health benefits to being fit. Being extremely overweight or obese brings with it obvious health problems. Although there is some debate over what constitutes a healthy BMI and how this is decided. However, it has now been recognised that the self-loathing that accompanies being unhappy with your body is also very detrimental to health. Some argue that it poses an even greater threat than the potential health problems of the extra pounds themselves. It seems as if avoiding the ever present temptations of unhealthy food in the 21st century can lead to a decline in mental and emotional wellbeing.

If you befriend your body you are likely to build a true regard and acceptance which in turn can result in looking after yourself rather than punishing yourself for not having the "right" body. Befriending your body is likely to lead to a more genuine awareness so, for example, understanding the relationship between hunger and food. And being in a position to question body image in terms of what "should" your own unique body look and feel like. And asking, according to who / compared to what?

In order for us to remain consumers of the body dissatisfaction markets, we must remain shamed and stigmatised. In order to provide those markets with a constant revenue stream, we must remain yoyo dieters who are "hungry" for the newest products and/or fighters of the signs of aging.

Denise Collins

Five
Food and movement

T he lifestyle we have in our modern advanced
21st century world is in many ways detrimental
to human beings. Human beings are evolved to
chase and catch, or toil, grow and harvest food. Now
we are offered ever more plentiful variety. We can
do our grocery shopping online and order takeaways
without even having to go outside or leave the
comfort of the sofa. We are creatures that over
thousands of years have evolved to eat whenever
food is available so that energy can be stored as fat to
protect us from times of famine. And we are evolved
to avoid unnecessary physical exertion in order to
conserve energy for chasing and producing food. Or
running away from or fighting predators. While
modern genetics play a small part, indeed scientists
have identified some gene mutations which make
certain people more likely to gain weight than
others, it is our general 21st century lifestyle and
changes in food consumption that are more likely to
be the reason many of us are getting fatter. Even in
the quite recent past our food was plainer, our
portions were smaller and we moved more. Special
occasion treats have now become everyday staples in
our diet, including such things as chocolate and

alcohol. The reduction in manual work, the growth of the use of labour-saving devices and technology, lots of screen time equals a more generally sedentary lifestyle for most. The explosion in consumption of processed "junk" food stuffs and the extensive use of refined sugar all contribute. Many processed "foods" consist of little more than fat, sugar and a cocktail of chemicals. These "foods" often have questionable nutritional value and are actually far removed from what could be considered to be real food. I personally experienced a good example of how far removed we have become from the notion of real food. After picking wild blackberries from a nearby meadow and harvesting apples from the trees in my garden, I was asked, "Are you sure they are safe to eat?"

We often do not appreciate that the food we buy pre-washed and packaged from the supermarket is laden with a cocktail of chemicals. Even "fresh meat", because livestock and poultry are given drugs to make them bigger and fatter. There appears to be evidence that consumption of the meat from these animals passes these drugs to us, which in turn make us fatter. Artificial sweeteners promised us calorie free options. Diet versions of foods and drinks can actually be more harmful than you might think. For example, drinking a diet, zero-calorie version of your favourite fizzy drink may seem like a health conscious choice. It provides a sweet fix minus the calories. However, some people argue that the artificial sweeteners that keep it calorie free, like aspartame, saccharin and sucralose, are dangerous. Artificial sweeteners have a more intense taste than sugar, so they can dull our senses to naturally sweet foods like fruit. Artificial sweeteners have been shown to have the same effect on your body as sugar; triggering insulin, which sends your body into fat storage mode and leads to weight gain.

Refined sugar is sweet, white and potentially lethal. I considered myself to be a reasonably intelligent person but my level of ignorance when it came to the relationship between sugar and being fat was astounding. I thought that sugar merely represented "empty" calories providing no nutritional value.

But it would seem the truth is far worse than that. Sugar is in fact more like a deadly, addictive poison that makes the body store fat because of its effects on our hormones and brain. Consuming sugar is like flipping a switch that tells your body to create and store fat. The way it does this is that sugar raises insulin levels; this tells the body to add to fat cells. It also makes the brain resistant to the hormone leptin. The result is that the brain doesn't recognise all the stored fat in the body so thinks it is in fact starving and so continues to create more fat. Could this begin to solve the mystery of why people become and stay fat, even if they are not eating really excessive amounts of food? It is not just the number of calories that you consume that is important. It is the effect that sugar has on the body and brain. I could go into what are good sugars and bad sugars, but I am no nutritionist so I would probably just complicate things unnecessarily. Essentially think: Sugar = instructing your body to store fat. As well as being a main ingredient in obvious sweet things, sugar is also hidden in all sorts of processed foods. This makes it difficult to avoid. The best place to make a start is to STOP eating the obvious sweet, sugary, man-made processed junk. This won't necessarily be easy because there is a lot of scientific evidence that sugar is addictive. It provides a release of opiates and dopamine in the reward system of the brain, the same areas stimulated by drugs like nicotine and cocaine. So basically you have to break the addiction in order to experience the benefits. If you do it will have a dramatic effect because basically your hormones will rebalance and your body will stop storing fat. If you don't you will not only stay fat but you will actually get fatter and fatter

Six

S o here are some ideas on how you can befriend
your body and improve body esteem:

1. Stop dieting. If diets worked you would only ever
    have to do one once. Recidivism or the tendency
    to relapse into previous undesirable types of
    behaviour is not merely odd examples of a few
    lapsed dieters being "naughty." It is not that you
    are bad, lack willpower, are weak or stupid. Diet
    industries are built on a foundation of shame and
    stigma, where dieters are eventually doomed to
    failure in order for the industry to make a profit.
    Stop obsessing about what you should or
    shouldn't, can or can't eat and create a normal
    relationship with food. Ditch the processed junk
    and eat real food when you are hungry. Stop
    when you have had enough. Learn to reconnect
    to your body so that you recognise the
    experiences of hunger and being satisfied and
    learn to understand your individual tastes and
    appetite. Food is fuel that should nourish your
    body. Reconnecting to natural intuitive eating
    will enable proper functioning of your
    metabolism, that series of processes by which
    food is converted into the energy and products
    needed to sustain life. Explore the reasons you

may eat when you are not hungry. What is the emotional hunger that you may be trying to satisfy with food?

2. Do not exercise. Just find opportunities to move more. The fitness and exercise industries are fantastic examples of creations which are designed specifically to solve a problem created by 21st century living. Our bodies are shaped by the physical activities we undertake. The less we physically move, the more our bodies reflect this fact and vice versa. In the 21st century most of us spend more and more time being less and less physically active. The fitness industry tries to sell us the idea that we can attain an aesthetic which, quite frankly, even if you spent your entire life in the gym, is unrepresentative of the majority of body shapes and types.

3. Develop an appreciation for what is right with your body. Your body is not all that you are, but it is you. You inhabit it. So to dis-identify and loathe it is an act of gross self-punishment. Find ways to cherish, admire, value and respect your body for the way it is rather than obsessing about the way you would rather it was.

4. Accept that you are going to get older and eventually die. Sorry to be the one to break that news to you but it is true. No matter how much you may resist, struggle or even fight, no matter

how many cosmetic surgery procedures, how much hair dye, how many hours you spend in the gym, or what kind of rejuvenating diet you have discovered. The natural progression of life is to mature, age and then shuffle off this mortal coil. It is the appropriate way of things. Rather than being depressing, acceptance of your own mortality and the life stage that you have reached can be very liberating. It can free you from the external pressures of attempting to hold back time and instead allow you to focus on greater meaning and purpose of existence. Psychologists have called this natural drive to fulfilment by various names, self-actualisation, individuation, etc. They talk about a growing curiosity about what comes next. After inevitable death, after physically ceasing to be. If you comfortably occupy the life stage you are at then you can begin to appreciate the type of wisdom accessible only from experience. You can discover and expand your core spiritual essence and the transient nature of this physical existence. This is not denial but matter-of-fact acceptance. When living true to your real authentic self you cannot be anything other than beautiful.

"I do not fear death. I had been dead for billions and billions of years before I was born, and had not suffered the slightest inconvenience from it."

- Mark Twain

A Few Conclusions On Befriending Your Body

Break away from the influence of the multi-billion pound and dollar industries created and dependent on you being unhappy with who you are. And instead begin to focus on the aspiration of true personal individual body esteem. The ideal image of what your physical appearance should be is, for the vast majority of people, always going to be unattainable. Therefore to pursue it is to be doomed to failure and misery. So instead of hating and punishing yourself for not being able to fit the "ideal", love and appreciate the body you have. The interesting thing is that what you focus on with kindness and appreciation tends to improve.

What Next?

I am sure you have noticed that during the safety briefing on an aircraft prior to takeoff passengers are instructed very clearly that in the event of an incident, "you must put your own oxygen mask on first before attempting to help anyone else". This is a great metaphor which illustrates that no one benefits in the long run if you try to help others but neglect yourself. Not only is it a simple truth that you cannot give when you have nothing to give, perhaps it goes even further than this. I believe that many people who focus on trying to help others are actually coming from a place of real deficit and lack which they try to address by focusing on attending to the needs of others. Without realising it consciously they help and give to others in the hope that someone will return the favour and in turn fill the void they have. Those people who do this would almost certainly be horrified at the suggestion that they are somehow engaging in a "giving to get" process because they genuinely believe they are giving to others while expecting and wanting nothing in return.

For all kinds of reasons it is deemed acceptable, even desirable, to show love, forgiveness and generosity to others. We are regarded as nice if we compliment others and put the needs of others before our own. The paradox is that while many people focus on loving, forgiving, being generous, complimenting and taking care of others, at the same time they engage in vicious self-criticism and are overly disapproving of themselves. They carry guilt and refuse to forgive themselves and do not merely neglect their own needs but sometimes actually engage in self-destructive behaviour and activities. It may be possible in the short term to ignore oneself and focus externally, but it is quite simply impossible to sustain this long term. No one can authentically maintain an external focus on others and neglect themselves for ever. Those who try burn out because they fail to understand why others do not act in similar altruistic ways. They feel resentful, depressed or get angry because no one returns the favour to them. The unconscious expectation is that if I put everyone before myself, others should do this for me. The truth is that if you expect, hope or seek someone else to fill the hole in your soul, you are doomed to disappointment.

Instead, begin to identify, address and look after your own needs. And find ways to start to direct compassion, love, forgiveness, nurturing and care towards you. Begin to practise self love, rather than hating or disapproving or looking for proof that you are always somehow in the wrong. Be generous to yourself, rather than unkind. Identify and take care of your own needs, rather than neglecting or, even worse, being cruel to yourself. Begin to find things to compliment yourself on, rather than constantly being critical. Develop practices that promote gratitude and appreciation for all that is good in your life, even the small things. Work on an approach of mindfulness, so that you can truly be in the present moment, rather than living in the past and getting lost in "if only". Rather than fearing, dreading or being anxious about the future and focusing on "what if?" I once read a quote that said no amount of guilt can change the past and no amount of anxiety can guarantee the future. The present moment is all that is real.

"How You Do Anything Is How You Do Everything"

Whether or not this statement is actually true is probably less important than the fact that it gets you thinking. What habits and patterns have you been running through the various spheres of your life?

Whatever goal, desire or ambition you have you can pretty much guarantee it will fit within one of the following categories. These are not listed in any particular order of importance. They are all important and each one impacts the others.

1. Money
2. Work
3. Relationships
4. Love
5. Health

6. Wellbeing
7. Spirituality; a search for purpose & meaning in life

Many people do not get what they really want because they do not go after what they really want. Instead they stay within their particular comfort zone. This is an interesting term because far from being comfortable that zone can be very restrictive and uncomfortable. I prefer the idea of a familiar zone, which may not actually be that comfortable but at least we are used to it!

Invitation. If you want to achieve more success, happiness and fulfilment in any or all of these areas of your life, I would like to extend my personal invitation to you; please get in touch with me to discover just how!

Let us have a quick preview of Money and Work. Now, many self-improvement books, courses and processes offer something along the lines of: ***"Let me show you how to get rich, be happy and have all of everything you ever really wanted"***.

Well, before I begin to help you on the road to making your fortune, I want to reveal something. I am not a millionaire. I do not own a helicopter or live a life of untold luxury and wealth in my own castle on a hilltop overlooking the ocean. I could, of course, tell you that I do and you would be none the wiser. If you believed me, you may be impressed, even envious. But the truth is that I don't even have a story about how I made millions and then lost or gave it all away and ended up living in my car. I am not going to tell you that you (too) can make millions with my secret system which is guaranteed to make you a financial success while you sleep. So why should you continue to read if I am not a millionaire?

Let me explain. I am a real person. I am quite ordinary really. I am a middle-aged, working class, white woman. My parents were not educated people, even though they were among the wisest I have ever met. In the past few years I have witnessed a multitude of "emperor's new clothes", "get rich quick" type schemes come and go. I have seen the most over-the-top shows of wealth from so-called gurus, which turned out to be merely illusions, usually built on lies. Or at the very least gross exaggeration and lots of credit. A nasty hangover from the 1980s and 1990s, "loads of money" culture where all that anyone wanted was to be rich beyond their wildest dreams. A time when the acquisition of expensive designer label stuff equated to personal success.

There were so many ways to get rich, buy to let property, becoming an entrepreneur business owner, playing the stock market etc. etc. none of which apparently required any talent or previous experience or knowledge.

Then I watched the pendulum swing the other way and everything became new-age, law of attraction, cosmic ordering where we were assured that we just needed to create a vision board, make a request (via reciting affirmations) to the universe and act "as if" we already had it. We were encouraged to "jump and the net will appear" in order to manifest abundance. And if this did not happen, the implication was we were not asking, visualising or wanting it hard enough.

As a result of all this hyperbole, I have realised something very enlightening. That the voice of the ordinary has become somehow remarkable and extraordinary. I like things that work. Call me pragmatic. I have had the great privilege to be in a professional position where I have had the opportunity to work with and on the links between our inner world of thoughts and feelings and the outer world we create as a result. I have worked with and studied the attitudes and mindsets of a great number of people. Both those who are successful and those who are not. I may not be a millionaire but I firmly believe that if making lots of money is truly what you want to achieve with your life then I can help you to do it.

Will owning this book guarantee it for you? Will even reading this book get it for you? No, of course it won't. The truth is that reward comes from the value you offer to others. You won't get rich just because you want to. You will get rich if others want to buy (and you decide to sell) what will help them. Gone for ever are the days of a job where a person is paid just for turning up. And financial success does not come from merely thinking about or desiring wealth. I do believe, however, that it is possible for you to discover your "golden egg". I believe there exists systems, ideas and tools that can assist you in becoming successful. This is essentially because success is a feeling, an attitude, a state of mind. One person's success is another's breadline. It is a perception, it is intangible. Does money guarantee you happiness, fulfilment, success? No, of course it doesn't. But neither does a lack of material wealth. Even the bohemians who reject materialist society require at least some cash sometimes! Money may not be the answer to all life's problems but it would be naive to think that a lack of money doesn't cause many of them.

Would you rather be rich or happy? Of course you can be both, but the first is of less value if you don't have the second. And many of those people who chase money are actually chasing the idea that if they had money they would be happy. But the one does not guarantee the other.

In the 21st century many of us have been fooled, perhaps by the grossly uneven distribution of wealth in developed countries, perhaps by the rise of celebrity culture where people are famous for being famous, that the fundamental principle of success and reward emanating from competence, skill and talent somehow no longer applies.

There is also the issue of suffering from a perceived lack based on the unrealistic, spurious images we are exposed to. The unreal expectations, the myth, the illusion which is little more than a joke, a con-trick played upon us, creating aspiration nations. Where we see things, lifestyles that others apparently enjoy and we will never have, but the mere fact that we can see them and know they exists means we feel entitled to the same. The world is full of people with potential. Most people miss out not because they are incapable but because they fail to do what needs to be done to get what they desire. The laws of cause and effect are simple and mostly very uncomplicated.

Many people could be successful at lots of things, but they bounce from one idea to another without investing the required amount of energy, time or effort to do it. It is like having a great recipe, buying all the ingredients and then leaving them sitting on the kitchen table and wondering why you are not enjoying the promised dish.

Many systems and schemes do actually provide solid sound information, but they omit vital elements. Which, to leave out, has the same result as buying a packet of seeds but paying no attention to the environment within which they are planted and wondering why they do not flourish. Being provided with the knowledge of what to do is one thing. But knowing how to take the required steps and how to apply what you know is something quite different.

Finance and career is an important area of life for all of us. The money we have (or don't have!) and the work we do (or would like to do) are central to the quality of our very existence. They can be either a significant source of fulfilment or dissatisfaction. During my research for this book it became apparent that although these two are linked, you could feel fulfilled in your career but still not earn enough money. Or you may do work that provides you with a good level of income but which does not satisfy you. Of course, if you are fortunate enough to do work you love and are passionate about and you earn enough money from it you might want to skip this section!

Why do I never have enough money?
or

Why am I stuck in a job I hate?
or

Why can't I get a job at all?

We could explore all the external reasons that exist in the 21st century for you experiencing one or more of the above problems.

We could discuss how there are over 2 million people who are unemployed in the UK at the time of writing this. We could examine the phenomena of entire families who have become trapped in patterns of deprivation, parents that have never worked having children who will never work, all seemingly doomed to an existence of surviving on state benefits and appearing on the *Jeremy Kyle Show*. We could talk about how many people are forced into working part-time because that is all they can get rather than because that's what they prefer, or those who can only get work on zero hour contracts because that is all employers are offering. We could point to the very changeable nature of work, where a job for life no longer exists and where children that are at primary school right now will grow up to undertake jobs that at this present moment do not even exist. We could look at the economy, interest rates, inflation or assess the true value of money.

We Could… But We Are Not Going To.

Instead I want to take a different approach to examining what is actually the problem. And to focus on seeking answers and solutions for you as a unique individual. This is important because I believe that you are much more powerful than perhaps you currently realise. And as the saying goes… with great power comes responsibility. So we are going to start with how you have created the situation you are currently in. Now, before you throw this book across the room in disgust that I could even suggest that your situation is in any way your own fault…

Please take a moment to consider the difference between the concepts of blame and responsibility. If you are to blame, this makes you guilty of something and if you are guilty then you are obviously in need of punishment! Not terribly useful in the context of improving the circumstances of your life. However, if you are responsible this makes you powerful and empowered to change things once you understand a little about why and how. Stick with me for a bit. I am on your side.

Let Us Take A Problem That Is VERY Common. For Example "The Problem Is That I Do Not Have Enough Money."

You could be forgiven for thinking that the solution to this problem is as simple as, "I just need some more." However, at least some of the reasons for the belief, "I do not have enough money" (and it is a belief, by the way, and not a fact, although if this is currently your situation you will most likely be living life as if it is a fact and not a belief!) are firmly rooted in 21st century living. To begin with let's examine the statement a little more closely: "The problem is that I do not have *enough* money." Enough for what exactly? And do you, in fact, know just how much enough would be? Anyone who has ever been in the situation of getting a pay rise to then very soon realise that the increase was *not enough,* understands that the question of what would be enough is far from straightforward.

Want Or Need?

Could it be that we have lost sight of the very real distinctions between what is a *want* and what is a *need*. What is something we would like and what is actually a necessity. Could it be that we have been hijacked by rampant consumerism and sold on the idea that we really need stuff that before we saw the advert we didn't even know existed? "If only I could win the lottery" has become a statement that apparently holds within it the answer to all of life's problems. That is, if you regard answers as having a price tag.

21ˢᵗ *Century Window On The World*

Before 24/7 multiple entertainment channels brought a window to a world we are not part of into our living rooms, before the advent of the internet, in the past we would only be exposed to levels of "prosperity" that we shared. Seeing worlds we are never likely to be part of (if, that is, you actually even believe what we are shown is in fact real) has created an undercurrent of discontent and dissatisfaction where *ordinary* has somehow become regarded as second rate, as not good enough. Is it that perhaps watching all those TV shows and peeking at others' glamorous lives via the internet has made us desire a life of celebrity, when we in fact work in a supermarket? There is, of course, nothing wrong with working in a supermarket. But if you do, do you really need as a necessity a designer handbag?

But Why Shouldn't I Have It?

This isn't about shoulds, or who deserve what. Life, apparently, isn't always fair. The point I am making is that it is all too easy, seductive in fact, in the 21st century to confuse not having enough with the inability to manage what you have got. There are various very simple universal principles that I wish to share with you in MMBB so that you can genuinely begin to design and create a life that you really want to live. MMBB is not a rainbows and unicorns, pixie dust and fairy wings approach that says you can have everything you want and you can have it right now without having to actually do anything. MMBB is about universal principles that are real.

And in order to improve anything it is first essential to become truly aware of the current situation. In this instance it means doing what you can, with what you have, rather than, for example, living beyond your means in an attempt to buy happiness on credit.

Doing Jobs We Hate In Order To Buy Stuff We Don't Need...

There is a great quote in the 1999 film *Fight Club* that goes "Advertising has us chasing cars and clothes. Working jobs we hate, so we can buy shit we don't need." If you are doing a job you truly hate you are likely to feel powerless to change things. The paradox is that even though you hate it you are probably also anxious that you might lose it. If you do not have a job at all you are likely to feel hopeless and helpless and look at the people working in the unemployment office and think, How on earth do they have a job and I don't?

The Need To Do Work That Is Meaningful And Makes A Positive Difference.

A good example of how money does not replace the desire to do work that has some higher purpose is provided by a book by Kevin Roose, *Young Money.* In order to write the book, Roose spent three years shadowing eight young Wall Street bankers. Although extremely well paid (Roose says that first year investment bankers make anywhere from $90,000 to $140,000, including yearend bonuses) he found that the majority were struggling with depression and health problems and expressed the desire to do something else.

British economist Roger Bootle has written about the difference between what he calls "creative" and "distributive" work. Creative work brings something new into the world that adds to the total available to everyone (e.g. a doctor treating patients, an artist producing art). Distributive work, on the other hand, is focused on beating the competition and winning the biggest share of a fixed-size market. Bootle explains, "There are some people who may derive active delight from the knowledge that their working life is devoted to making sure that someone else loses, but most people do not function that way. Most people like to have a sense of worth, and that sense usually comes from the belief that they are contributing to society".

Unless it is somehow possible to either find or create some greater significance for the work we do, beyond getting paid, we are likely to be resentful and dissatisfied. If the work we do is merely a way to fund our life, the need for more and more materially is likely to escalate. While not all occupations provide an intrinsic sense of purpose, accomplishment or pride, it is possible to affirm that you are doing a particular job out of choice rather than because you have to. This decision is in itself empowering. There is a story that goes: during a visit to the NASA Space Center in 1962, President Kennedy noticed a maintenance man. Kennedy is said to have asked, 'What do you do around here?' 'Well, Mr. President,' the maintenance man replied, 'I'm helping put a man on the moon'. Now whether this story is actually true or not is beside the point. It serves to exemplify the notion that if we can find or create meaning in our work that is personally motivating it is possible to be inspired and happy doing any job.

The sense of having choices is essential to human happiness. During financially tough times in my earlier life I found myself undertaking a variety of menial jobs in order to make ends meet. However, I always focused on the real "why" I was doing the job... even if it was simply because I needed the money I always reminded myself I had options. I had choices. I chose to do the job because I wanted the money to feed my kids or to pay for education in order to ultimately improve our situation. So I found some greater meaning to working which helped me so that even in a horrible job I decided it was better than not working. Also, rather than spreading resentment and misery at "having to do such a horrible job" I would consciously seek out ways to make small positive differences to people I came into contact with. Simple and sometimes somewhat random acts of kindness made intolerable situations somehow more tolerable. These attitudes of mind put me in control of my life. I was thus empowered even when situations were challenging. The truth is we do all have choices. When we say we have no choice, what we really mean is that we do not like the choices we have and we wish we had a different one.

Identifying and understanding the deficits in your life that money cannot provide a solution for and beginning to address these directly can be wonderfully liberating. MMBB is a system that illustrates how our thoughts and feelings can be influenced by our environment, in much the same way as seeds will either grow or die depending on the soil in which they are planted. It is therefore essential to pay attention to your environment and make changes as appropriate. Our thoughts and feelings constitute our inner world and it is in fact our inner world which dictates our experience of the outer world. Our thoughts and feelings determine how we perceive external events and how we react emotionally. What we think and feel will determine the actions we take and how we behave and these in turn create the results we get, which we then in turn experience via thoughts and feelings. And so the cycle goes on.

A great place to start is where you are. It is difficult to plot a journey to somewhere you want to go until you ascertain your current location. So start where you are with what you have. Assess the reality of your situation. Explore how things really are.

Don't catastrophise and think it is all bad or make it worse than it actually is. But don't put on the rose tinted glasses of positive thinking either and see your life as all wonderful and better than it is. Take a good long hard look at things as they really are for you right now. Then consider what it is that you actually want that you think money or a different job will give to you. Ask people what having more money would mean to them and they usually give variations of one of two responses: either security or freedom. Whichever response they give provides insight into what they consider they currently lack in life.

Whatever your story so far, good bad of indifferent, where you are, what you have or don't have is the result of the thoughts, feelings and actions you have taken or not taken. Every choice every decision is part of a cause and effect response. You are already getting results. They just may not be the results you would like. You are already powerful. You are already in control of steering the direction of your life. Even if you did not realise it. You are in the driver's seat and if you didn't realise that, then every action and reaction, every choice and decision will have consequences that you have not planned. This is why it can seem as if life just happens to you. In reality, there are no coincidences. We live in a universe that is responding to us even if we are unaware of it.

Before I wind up this little tome, I would like to offer you a parting gift. Here is a fairly simple, step by step formula to assist with effective problem solving, better decision making and fulfilling your full potential. Of course, simple is not necessarily the same as easy, so if you want help to work on getting more of what you want in your life, please respond to the invitation. I hope to meet you in person very soon.

An 11 Step All-Purpose Success Formula

1. Identify and acknowledge any emotional / mental / physical / spiritual discomfort. Rather than struggling with it, fighting it, trying to avoid it, mask it or distract yourself from it, realise that no discomfort has to prevent you from taking the right action.

2. Focus on the present. Rather than dwelling on the past and what has happened or attempting to predict the future and what may or may not happen. Assess the reality of your current situation. Make a distinction between what is within your influence and what is outside of what you can influence. (I once heard someone

say that "control is an illusion, influence is the best we can hope for"!)

3. Realistically define the problem or challenge or change that you want to implement. Define what you actually have right now without making it seem better or worse than it actually is.

4. Realistically define your desired outcome. In other words, what do you want instead of what you have? I consciously use the word realistically because although I may believe that "anything is possible", you need to start where you are with what you have in order to avoid becoming overwhelmed and disheartened. Assessing the current conditions enables you to make progress step by step. There is no point in setting a desired outcome of winning the next London marathon if you can't yet even jog to the end of the road. The gap between steps 3 and 4 represents a choice point where positive change is possible

5. Separate information / evidence / facts from feelings, hunches or beliefs. Then sort these into: relevant to the situation,
Irrelevant to the situation
And drama/smokescreen (which are feelings / concerns that are neither relevant nor irrelevant to the situation). And focus only on what is relevant to the situation. It is not that the other

things are not important. They are just not relevant.

6. Based on all of the above explore all the possible, potential options that exist to get from where you are to where you want to be.

7. Objectively assess the pros and cons of each option.

8. Once you have done this, choose an option. Even if the choices available are not perfect you need to make a choice in order to start to take action.

9. Identify potential obstacles that might prevent success. The purpose of this is not to put you off that option but to enable you to develop a contingency plan. To allow you to consider ways you will potentially overcome any obstacles if they do occur.

10. Make a plan of the required action in the following way. Start at the end as if you were at the point of having already achieved the desired result and work backwards. That way you can decide what needs to be done when. Look at the following time-frames: what needs to be done right away, immediately? What needs to be done in the short, medium and longer term?

11. Do. Take action. Get started. Then follow the DRD process = Do Review Do.

Do = take action. Review = if what you are doing is working, continue. If it is not working, do something else. When you have achieved your desired outcome, decide on the next one. Do = because you are never done until you're dead.

Conclusion and an invitation

As I write this there is increasing unrest, violence and sectarian extremism across the world, which did make me wonder if the words in this book seem by comparison somewhat petty. On reflection, however, I believe that each one of us, in some small way, can make a positive difference in defeating the ignorance and fear to spurn such atrocities. Even if we can only do this one person at a time. I believe the world would be a better place if each and every person took responsibility for their own success and happiness

Cruelty, hatred and brutality can never be justified. They can never be right. No matter in whose name atrocities are committed. To violently overpower another in order to make them convert to the same way of thinking can never be sustainable. No matter how big, strong or powerful a person, a race or a regime is it is merely a matter of time until they themselves become the victims. So in the end everyone loses. Violence, terror and hatred create a path that leads to eventual destruction of the body, mind and the spirit for everyone, so in the end no one wins. The only path to true freedom and peace is acceptance and love. Anything else is an insidious poison that will be the downfall of everyone, including those who think they are winning at any particular point in the game.

A good friend of mine said that he believed the answer to all negativity is simply; to love, to be loved and to learn. To love is to give, to be loved is to accept, to learn enables expansion, reflection and, as a result, choice.

The purpose of this book is to spread the idea that by mastering your mind and befriending your body you can become who you were always meant to be. As Oscar Wilde said, "Be yourself because everyone else is taken." You do not have to fit some standard ideal; instead you can become the very best version of yourself possible. And you can do this by rising above others who might hold you down, rather than trampling on anyone else in order to ascend higher.

Invitation. If you want to be part of an ultimate healing, transformation experience I would like to invite you to make contact to discover how.

www.masteryourmindbefriendyourbody.co.uk

About the author Denise Collins MSc. BSc. (Hons)

Denise is the founder and principal of *The Hummingbird Effect Academy*. A successful therapist and coach, she has been designing and delivering NLP, Coaching, Hypnotherapy, professional and personal development courses since 2005. Born into a working class family, she left school with few qualifications. She got married for the first time aged 18 had a child at 20 and was a single parent living on state benefits by the age of 21. During a heart to heart with her father, she revealed her dismay at what a failure she was. He told her to stop feeling sorry for herself and "go and do an evening class or something". This conversation prompted her to embark on what became an enduring love affair with adult education, self-improvement and overcoming adversity. She worked in voluntary and paid capacities in various helping organisations, including adult literacy schemes, victim support, Samaritans, Relate, projects to help inner city youth and underage mums, those caring for people with life limiting conditions and women facing unplanned pregnancy. Her qualifications now include: an MSc in Coaching Psychology from The University of East London, an upper second honours degree BSc in Social Sciences from South Bank University, an RSA Teaching & Learning in Adult Education, an Open University management studies certificate, a Diploma in analytical and cognitive hypnotherapy and psychotherapy, NLP practitioner, master practitioner and trainer, certified by NLP co-creator John Grinder. Denise has been married to her "current" husband John since 1986. In 1992 they moved from London to Essex. They have three grown-up offspring, two grandchildren and three dogs.

Denise says, *"I believe the world is full of people who fulfil only a fraction of their true potential. My desire is to help people discover who they really are, what their purpose is and how they can become the best version of their own unique self possible."*

www.masteryourmindbefriendyourbody.co.uk

www.hummingbirdeffect.com